INTERMITTENT FASTING FOR WOMEN OVER 50

A GUIDE TO HELP YOU WIN THE BATTLE AGAINST
WEIGHT LOSS. THIS BOOK WILL HELP YOU RESET
YOUR METABOLISM, LOSE WEIGHT AND REACH YOUR
BODY'S FULL POTENTIAL TO LOOK AND FEEL GREAT

MARIA LIMON

CONTENTS

INTRODUCTION

It's not like 50 is the new 30. It's like 50 is the new chapter."

— SHARON STONE

When Dolly Parton was asked, "What do you want people to say about you a hundred years from now?" she replied: "Well, I want them to say, 'Doesn't she look good for her age?'"

Isn't it true that age is simply a number? Having said that, it is a significant number in our life. It's a unique number that should be treasured and loved.

From the delight of grandkids to the bittersweet sense of retirement, there are many adjustments to contemplate and negotiate during this chapter in your life. One of the most noticeable changes around this age is a woman's health starting to speed towards increasingly unexpected and occasionally frightening bodily changes.

Is intermittent fasting truly "the one?" there is no magical formula or guide that can indeed turn back the clock, and numerous claims have been made via books and seminars that all claim to be "the one." This book will not make misleading promises or provide you with a shortcut to the fountain of youth. It will provide you with a proven and proper strategy that has been used and endorsed by millions of people all over the globe who want to feel younger, reduce stubborn belly fat, and have the energy to live a fulfilled life rather than get by.

This book personalizes intermittent fasting material to women in their fifties and beyond. No stones will be unlifted; the good, bad, and ugly facts regarding the different ways of intermittent fasting will be documented for you to digest, along with recipes and fitness ideas to help you on this fascinating trip.

Every one of us has attempted a 'diet' at least a few times and a fancy new 'how to appear younger' cosmetic trend. The issue is that it always seems to be a band-aid solution. You may have seen some benefits in the shape of a few pounds gone, but this is never something you can maintain over a long period of time.

The information in this book is supported by the setbacks I and so many others have had on the road to weight reduction, as well as learnings from many clients about what they needed to do to eventually remain on track and not tap out every now and then, wasting all the hard work.

Failure is usually due to a lack of tools to keep you on track, which can ultimately alter your whole perspective toward the objectives you want to attain. Motivation quickly leads to despair, then BOOM! You've returned to square one.

Women in America have a higher life expectancy than males, meaning they may develop long-time health issues as they age. So, as you approach your 50s and beyond, be aware of a few of the health-related obstacles you are more vulnerable to and know how to give yourself the most incredible opportunity of navigating them (don't worry, no physical hurdling is needed of you in any of the intermittent fasting programs!) Reading this book will challenge your mentality, help you plan out your objectives, and provide you with a comprehensive overview of the benefits and drawbacks of intermittent fasting, as well as information on how to accelerate sustainable weight reduction via exercise and cooking.

It may surprise you to learn that your body is as conscious of the stage of life you are entering as your family and friends who may have spent months planning that substantial 50th or 60th celebration. If you haven't prepared your body and health for this new point in life, it's not too late to make a dramatic, safe, and revolutionary shift with the intermittent fasting advice you will find in this book.

The notion of intermittent fasting is relatively simple, versatile, and applicable to any lifestyle. A significant research published in 2019 reduced intermittent fasting to 'you adjusting your eating pattern and splitting it into periods of eating and fasting.' In layman's words, you will create a weekly timetable in which you will have a period when you have no food and a period immediately after that where you may consume food. Isn't it simple?

There are four well-known eating patterns in intermittent fasting, each with its own set of meal plans. This book will teach you about various eating regimens and how they function, so you can determine which one is ideal for you.

The conventional wisdom that establishes intermittent fasting as a kind of self-starvation is entirely false. According to several studies, our bodies can survive for weeks without eating before we start "starving." Is this a recommendation to fast for long periods of time? Absolutely not! The idea is to demonstrate that, regardless of how we feel when we don't consume food, our bodies can be more than able to adjust, even in severe conditions such as not eating for weeks.

There is an obligation to abstain from eating while fasting intermittently; regrettably, there is no way around it. The purpose of this is not to punish your body; instead, it is to generate a calorie deficit. Some programs may recommend 24 hours of no eating, while others may just require 13 hours, with both alternatives possibly being as effective as the other. These alternatives are based on numerous aspects, such as what food you consume during your feasting window. This should prove that, despite any hunger pangs, your body will adjust and prosper.

One of the primary reasons why an aging body's health starts to degrade outside of biology and the inevitable decline we can all anticipate is that we have become used to our bodies controlling what and when we eat. No, your body will not like it at first! But then, your body will begin to accept and adapt to what you instruct it to do.

Many of us are guided by our body's desire rather than our necessity, and the two are readily confused. When we have a poor day, for example, our body tells us that we need to overindulge in food and drinks that our bodies don't truly need, and we don't feel any better as a result. Most people have lost control of their bodies, and the consequences of this lack of discipline and focus can be seen in health deterioration, weight concerns, and so many other aspects of our life. Intermittent fasting is a method that may help you regain control of your body and break the pattern of power that your body has over you.

With a systematic strategy for a new eating routine, you will regain control of the direction of your body type, health, and emotional well-being. Your body will oppose this shift because it is used to determine what, when, and how you eat. Our bodies have been indulged for many years with little discipline or structure. Our bodies may kick and scream, weep and stamp their figurative feet at the start of this regulated eating schedule because it is not receiving what it believes we need and is no longer in control- you are. You will be via intermittent fasting.

Intermittent fasting provides more advantages than you may think, besides reducing weight and maintaining shape. While you may be solely thinking about the weight reduction advantages, intermittent fasting also has physical and mental health benefits. Intermittent fasting improves muscle and joint health, decreases depression, reduces your risk of illnesses such as heart disease, cancer, diabetes, and metabolic disorders, and lowers blood sugar and insulin levels.

Our bodies are intelligent, adaptable, and, most importantly, unique. When it comes to successful weight reduction or health improvement procedures, each individual's biological make-up is different and necessitates a distinct strategy. This is why most diets work for a few weeks before your body adjusts and your results stagnate.

We will also look at recipes that mainly target aspects of your health that you want to enhance, such as skin care, mental health, energy, and so much more. Is this method of weight reduction acceptable for the majority of people? Absolutely.

There are several exceptions due to pre-existing health issues, medicine, and other factors, but all of this will be addressed and described in the early chapters. With this book's help, you can pick from many recipes and intermittent fasting regimens to mold and shape your desired end.

Whether it's on your taste senses or your physique, enjoyment doesn't have to end at fifty. You can still eat delicious, nutritious meals while looking as youthful as you want. Do you want to make intermittent fasting a way of life as you enter your fifties? Do you want to know how to do it? Continue reading!

1

AGING, WOMEN, AND WEIGHT LOSS - THE CONNECTIONS

The assumption that the functions of a woman's body are meant to produce misery and anguish and that women need a considerable lot of medical care and testing to remain healthy is one of the antiquated core notions dominating our health care system. In truth, our creator created the female body as a source of pleasure, reproduction, movement, energy, and well-being. Though this is undoubtedly the reality of many women, there is another, better way.

Our bodies are linked to the moon, waves, and seasons. We are created to thrive. We, the human race, have arrived at a fork in the road, a tipping point when old, outdated beliefs and habits are collapsing all across the world. The present healthcare crisis is only one illustration of this breakdown that I am all too acquainted with. There is no need to be afraid of the old collapsing since it makes room for new, more sustainable, but also healthier systems and ideas to emerge in all facets of the human experience on Earth, along with how we deal with the experience of living in a female body.

Instead of merely waiting for sickness to strike, it can flourish in a female body. It all comes down to this: despite our specific situations, histories, or ages, we all have the inner direction that we can listen to in order to generate flourishing health right now. We are born with this inner direction, which manifests as feelings and wants that steer us toward (and away from) things that feel good and are suitable for us and away from things that feel unpleasant and are harmful to us. It's as easy as that. Love, pleasure, contentment, and health are hardwired into our DNA.

Though we were frequently talked out of our ambitions as youngsters, I've learned that we may trust the impulses that motivate us to get out of bed in the morning. Our aspirations are the conduits through which the healing life energy flows and fills our bodies. They are what make life worthwhile to live. They are the foundation of our aspirations and dreams. And they inevitably carry the secrets to curing our bodies and our whole lives.

WOMEN AND THE AGING PROCESS

When asked how old you are, you most likely respond regarding the number of years since birth. That is your chronological age. However, your doctor may suggest you have the physical fitness of a 21-year-old. Depending on how many decades previously you were born, this is your biological age.

Your chronological age will always be a fixed number. However, your biological age is determined by various elements that might vary regularly. The distinction between the two may be startling and warrants additional investigation.

What exactly is chronological aging?

Your chronological age is the length of time between your birth and the stated date. It's your age in years, weeks, days, and so on. This is how most people describe their age. It's also a significant risk factor for chronic illnesses, death, and impairments in body functioning like hearing and memory.

What exactly is biological aging?

The main principle behind biological aging is that aging happens gradually as damage to different cells and tissues in the body accumulates. Biological age, also known as biological or functional age, is different from chronological age because it considers more factors than just the day you were born.

The exact figure is determined by several biological factors and physiological development parameters. Some examples are:

- Genetics of chronological age (for instance, how fast your body's antioxidant shields start working).
- Diseases and other disorders are caused by lifestyle nutrition.
- Medical practitioners may determine what age your body performs like by using these principles and numerous mathematical models.

Chronological age is an important consideration. However, it is not always synchronized with the biological age. For instance, if you're a 29-year-old person who doesn't exercise, exclusively eats high-fat meals, and has smoked two packs of cigarettes each day for the previous ten years, you're likely to be older than 29.

So, if biological age is a stronger predictor of how well you age, how can you precisely measure it?

Methylation plays an essential role in numerous bodily functions. Less or more methylation may have a negative impact on many elements of your health and life. A recent study (Mindikoglu, 2022) indicates that DNA methylation is essential in health and aging. In recent years, researchers have discovered a relation between the aging of various physiological organs and the degree of DNA methylation - dubbed "epigenetic clocks."

The magnitude to which locations of your DNA consist of methyl groups – indicating that they are "methylated" – can be impacted not only by age but also by a variety of biological and environmental factors such as your nutrition, physical health, microbiome, psychological health, as well as environmental factors such as cigarette smoke and other pollutants.

Telomere length is another biomarker connected with age and health. Telomeres are proteins present at the ends of chromosomes that safeguard the function and structure of DNA. Shorter telomeres are linked to worse health and older biological age. Even though telomeres naturally deteriorate and shrink with time, research suggests several variables may hasten this process. Some variables, like heredity, are uncontrolled; however, you can regulate other factors that contribute to telomere shortening, such as:

- Obesity
- Poor Diet
- Fewer hours of sleep
- Lack of exercise
- Smoking

We are still a long way from learning all there is to know about DNA methylation, telomeres, or aging. Although research into the underlying processes is still in its early stages, much is known about how to remain healthy. For instance, are DNA methylation and telomere length directing the aging process, or are they just markers?

CHANGES THAT YOUR BODY GOES THROUGH AS YOU BECOME OLDER

Here is what happens to a woman's body as she becomes older:

Body Weight

Both men and women gain weight as they become older. Your body does not burn calories as efficiently as it did when you were in your twenties or teens. It happens when metabolism and muscular growth slow down. Men, on the other hand, may have it a bit easier.

Males' bodies tend to cease storing a lot of fat by the moment they reach the age of 55, while it simply continues on and on for females till the day they die. The majority of the fat is stored on the hips before menopause. They may also be systemic, which implies they only exist under the skin.

Women may begin to gain abdominal and belly fat after menopause. It is hazardous since it grows near crucial organs. It may raise the risk of chronic illnesses like:

- Heart problems
- Diabetes
- High blood pressure

Skin and Hair Health

Your skin might become dry, fragile, and thin as you age. All of these factors contribute to a quicker loss of skin moisture and suppleness, resulting in wrinkles and fine lines. Years of sun tanning or staying out in the sun for an extended period of time may cause wrinkles, dehydration, age spots, and sometimes even cancer. Scratches, wounds, and bruises could also occur.

The same thing might happen to your hair. This might explain why you have increased hair loss as you get older. Your skin and hair will change as you age. It does not matter if you like this or not.

Cardiovascular Health

Weight gain and hormones after 50 are not the only side effects of aging. There's also cardiovascular health to consider. According to observational studies, estrogen reduction may raise the risk of heart disease in menopausal women.

Other studies suggest that estrogen may protect blood vessels, especially arteries, from injury. It might also influence the inflammatory response. Women may be able to lower their risk of cardiovascular disease by following a healthy diet, exercising regularly, and avoiding smoking.

Cognitive Health

The aging process may also influence a gender's susceptibility to age-related memory loss, including neurodegenerative disorders like Alzheimer's and dementia.

According to a 2016 study, males are more likely than women to develop age-related cognitive deterioration. According to a 2019 research, women may be more susceptible to Alzheimer's than males.

The cause is stress. According to a 2018 research published in Frontiers in Neuroscience, alteration in female hormones may influence autophagy. Autophagy, for those who are unfamiliar, refers to the body's capacity to eliminate damaged cells while regenerating new ones.

Cellular Health

Your chronological and biological ages do not have to be the same. Your birth certificate may show that you are 50 years old, but your body is either 60 or 40 years old.

Many explanations have been proposed to explain these developments. The free radicals, as well as reactive oxygen species (ROS) hypothesis, is one of them. The distinction is due to differences in cellular health (or your cells). Free radicals are unstable chemicals that may harm cells, particularly the mitochondria, which provide energy and play an essential role in metabolism. ROS may be produced by cells, although they do not cause significant damage thanks to antioxidants.

Antioxidant levels, on the other hand, decrease as you age. Oxidative stress occurs when the body has much more free radicals than antioxidants. What does this have to do with women? Some studies connect estrogen production stoppage to oxidative stress.

Another possibility is concerned with telomere length. Telomeres are the DNA caps located at the ends of chromosomes. Short telomeres may be caused by factors like genetic susceptibility, pollution, and chemicals. They may also get shorter when cells divide.

Telomere shortening may cause aging and senescent tissues. These are cells that are unable to divide. Some research suggests that lifestyle adjustments, such as weight management, may help to prolong or lengthen telomeres.

Risk of Chronic and Serious Diseases

Osteoporosis, cancer, urinary inconsistency, and migraine headaches are some of the other chronic illnesses that could happen right after turning 50.

Osteoporosis, a disorder in which the bones get brittle, is one of the age-related illnesses associated with a high risk of death. Even a simple fall may endanger one's life. Because your body grows density quickly while you're young, you feel powerful. On the other hand, the aging process may begin to slow down by the age of 30.

A bone density test is generally included in health programs for women over the age of 50. Because of considerable hormonal changes, you reduce bone density quicker between 35 and menopause. Your doctor may advise boosting your calcium and vitamin D consumption when required.

These two operate together to help the immune system and improve mineral absorption, strengthening bones. The doctor may also advise modest physical or low-impact exercise such as walking, which should be supplemented with strength training.

Throughout one woman's life, her breasts undergo several modifications. They get engorged with milk during pregnancy. Estrogen levels decrease as you age and menopause occurs. It might cause the breasts to sag or droop.

Breast cancer is possibly the most severe threat to breast health. It may develop as a result of both gene mutation and changes in estrogen levels. According to research, continuous exposure to the hormone may raise cancer risk. These possibilities include the following:

- Menstruating at an early age
- Experiencing menopause at a later age
- Taking menopausal hormone treatment (MHT) tablets to control menopausal symptoms

Older individuals at risk for breast cancer may consider getting a mammography before age 50. Learning how to reduce estrogen naturally may also assist in reducing the hazards.

Urinary incontinence is the inability to regulate one's bladder. You may have already peed before entering the bathroom. Pelvic organ prolapse is a frequent cause of this illness. The muscles and ligaments that keep the organs together, such as the bladder, might weaken or become loose. Pelvic organ prolapse may be exacerbated by childbirth and hormonal changes.

Migraine frequency is greatly influenced by shifting sex hormone levels in women throughout menstruation and during the menopausal transitions. While migraine usually improves after menopause, perimenopause may be linked with considerable deterioration in incidence and symptoms, owing to variable estrogen levels.

Aging is characterized by continual, progressive, and natural changes. Many bodily functions progressively diminish throughout early middle age. The age of 65 is considered the start of old age. According to history, the retirement age is 65, although several factors for premature aging have been seen throughout the last few generations.

Let us remind ourselves once more:

- A person's chronological age is the number of years they have lived. It has little relevance in terms of health. The primary cause of body weight fluctuation in the elderly is age-related health issues and loss of functioning.

- The variations in the body that occur as humans age are referred to as biological age. However, it affects some individuals sooner than others, with some becoming old at the age of 65 and others not becoming old for a decade.
- Psychological age influences how individuals react to various circumstances and events.

Typical aging results in regular internal changes related to age and environment; nevertheless, some of these changes may be aberrant. Few changes are unexpected and undesirable, but they result from the aging process.

Healthy aging refers to preventing and delaying the negative consequences of aging. It is gained through eating a balanced and nutritious diet, exercising regularly, and being intellectually engaged.

Body form changes are typical as people age, but they may be delayed by living a healthy lifestyle. The human body comprises lean tissue (muscle plus organs), bones, water, and fats. Fat builds up in the body. Some cells in the muscles, kidneys, liver and other body organs are lost as we age.

After the age of 30, body fat progressively grows, with a one-third fat differential between young and elderly.

Fat builds up in the center of the body and across the internal organs. Changes in body form caused by extra fat, leg muscles, or stiffer joints may make it harder to move, leading to falls and fractures.

Males and women have various variations in body weight; around the age of 55, men tend to acquire weight and then progressively lose weight because testosterone levels in male sex hormones decrease with age.

Fats take the place of lean muscular tissue. Women put on weight until the age of 65, then progressively lose weight. Part of the weight reduction comes later on.

Because of the impact on lifestyle choices, the aging process occurs swiftly. Age-related physical changes, on the other hand, may be minimized. Regular exercise, a balanced diet rich in fruits and vegetables, healthy fats, whole grains, and alcohol in moderation helps prevent difficulties.

AGING AND WEIGHT GAIN

Weight increase, which leads to obesity, is a significant hazard to the health of the elderly. According to the World Health Organization, around 2.3 billion older adults are overweight, while 700 million are obese

(WHO). Obesity is classified as a chronic condition that affects people of all ages.

Most elderly persons in the medium and upper socioeconomic classes are prone to obesity due to sedentary lives and limited physical exercise.

Obesity is regarded as a significant risk factor for noncommunicable diseases (NCDs). Compared to weight reduction in Australia, the weight gain proportion increases with age.

Obesity arises when calorie intake exceeds caloric expenditure. The body contributes to increasing body fat till the age of 62, between the ages of 50 and 65. Hormonal changes occur around age 65, causing a fat buildup in the body.

Changes in environmental factors are also contributing to a rise in obesity among the elderly. Healthy habits are difficult to follow when food eating habits shift from traditional to contemporary and regular exercise routines fade.

Genes, age, gender, lifestyle, family traditions, culture, rest, and even where you live and work may all impact your weight. Some of these variables might make maintaining or achieving a healthy weight difficult. Following a healthy eating pattern, including exercising consistently, on the other hand, may assist in maintaining your body as fit as possible as you age.

Metabolism, or how the body obtains energy from meals, might vary as we age. This implies that some older people may need to become more active or consume fewer calories to maintain or attain their target weight.

Other elderly folks may unwittingly lose weight. This may occur if you lose your appetite, have difficulties leaving home to get food, have discomfort while chewing or ingesting, or forget to eat.

Maintaining a healthy weight is a crucial component of aging well. Elevated body mass index (BMI) in older individuals, like in earlier stages of life, might raise the probability of developing health issues. Heart disease, high blood pressure, stroke, and diabetes are examples. These hazards may be reduced by losing weight or weight maintenance.

Being underweight raises your risk of getting health issues. If you have a low BMI, you are more prone to develop medical problems such as osteoporosis and anemia, and recovering from a sickness or infection may be more difficult.

Being physically active and eating nutritious foods may help you maintain or reach a healthy weight, feel more energized, and reduce your risk of developing various health issues. Eating nutritious meals and getting at least 150 minutes of physical exercise every week is essential.

Calories are the units of measurement for the energy your body obtains from the foods and beverages you ingest. To maintain your current weight, your body requires a particular amount of calories every day, which varies based on your activity level and other variables. Exercise more or consume fewer calories than suggested to lose weight. Increase your calorie intake while maintaining moderate exercise to acquire weight.

This book's theme would mean combining a potent diet program with specific activities and going about it consistently. The truth is that regardless of age, there is just one way to lose unnecessary weight and maintain an average, healthy weight—and that is to combine good nutrition with regular exercise. You'll learn about these exercises later in the book. Still, starting with the next chapter, you'll familiarize yourself with intermittent fasting, a weight control method that's safe and effective for you even in your 50s.

Intermittent fasting has grown in popularity in recent years owing to its many health advantages and the fact that it does not limit your dietary options. Studies show that fasting boosts metabolism and psychological health and perhaps prevents various malignancies. It may help protect against particular muscle, nerve, and joint diseases that often affect women over the age of 50. Let's go to Chapter 2 and learn all we can about this style of food consumption.

Self-assessment Test:

1. Where are you now? Determine your target or ideal weight based on conventional weight-to-height ratio and factoring in age as well. Based on what's learned throughout the chapter, make a self-assessment to determine your current state of health and fitness and where you want or need to be.
2. What number would you give your overall habits of eating healthy foods?
3. How many times do you exercise per week?

THE BASICS OF INTERMITTENT FASTING

Fasting is a way of life for many people. And intermittent regularly implies a broken cyclic pattern. The theory behind this sort of dieting or lifestyle modification is to establish a calorie deficit and stimulate the body to use stored fats for energy, resulting in healthy and long-term fat reduction.

Intermittent fasting is a thriving lifestyle adjustment that significantly benefits those practicing it. Intermittent fasting has been shown to help with anything from curing diabetes and thyroid issues to offering relief from life-threatening cancers.

HOW DOES INTERMITTENT FASTING WORK?

Unlike other weight loss solutions, intermittent fasting is reasonably simple to implement. It is not a kind of dieting. Intermittent fasting is a way of living that leaves you more energized and full of life, allowing you to enjoy every waking minute of your day and get a decent night's sleep when you eventually call it a day.

Intermittent fasting has grown in popularity due to the ease with which it is possible to fast and get health advantages. Intermittent fasting comes in several forms, such as 16:8, and 5:2, alternate day fasting, eat stop eat, and so on.

In layman's terms, intermittent fasting entails eating for a certain amount of time throughout the day and fasting the rest of the time. In 16:8, intermittent fasting, for example, the eating window is 8 hours and the fasting period is 16 hours. It may seem to be an impossible feat when you read 16 hours of fasting. But what if I told you that out of the 16 hours of fasting, you'd sleep for 8-10 hours? That leaves just 6-8 hours of awake time, during which you will be unable to eat. But don't be concerned!

When you follow the 16:8 intermittent fasting schedule, your next meal occurs at noon the following day. Water and other zero-calorie liquids, such as black coffee, are permitted during this time. Assume you eat your meal around 8:00 pm. You finish your day and wind down about 11 pm after supper. When you wake up at 6 or 7 am the following day, you will have been fasting for 11 hours. Isn't it incredible? You need to train your body for a few more hours without food! Let us go further and learn the fundamentals of intermittent fasting!

THE FUNDAMENTALS OF INTERMITTENT FASTING

- This is the most basic and straightforward approach to dieting.
- Unlike several other diets that need tracking macro and micronutrient consumption, intermittent fasting does not necessitate keeping track of any of these parameters.
- There are no limits on ingesting any dietary categories or specific foods on their own. However, eating nutritious, wholesome, home-cooked meals is recommended to get the most out of an intermittent fasting regimen. Avoiding junk food in all forms is preferable.
- Some of the healthier food types that may be included in an intermittent fasting diet include

leafy greens, fresh fruits, nuts, dried fruits, poultry, and lean meat.

- Avoid CAFO meats and conventionally contaminated veggies. Instead, choose grass-fed beef and organic veggies.
- Intermittent fasting should be done slowly and steadily. It is best to avoid making significant changes in a short period of time. For example, you could fast for 20 hours straight on the first day of intermittent fasting. Such extreme measures will do more damage than good. To be successful and get the advantages of intermittent fasting, you must allow your body time to adjust to the fasts. Begin with fasting for 12-14 hours and work your way up.
- Always with your doctor or a nutritionist before initiating a fast or making substantial modifications to your fasting pattern.
- To stay hydrated, drink water and no-calorie beverages at regular intervals. Caffeine may be used during the fasting period, although it is best to restrict caffeine consumption for various reasons, including minimizing acid reflux and dehydration.
- Exercise is an essential component of every diet regimen. Exercise is as vital as, if not more important than, what you eat. A balanced

approach to intermittent fasting requires light exercise and increased daily physical activity.

- Aside from exercising, a regular sleep routine is essential. Sleeping and getting up at the same time every day provides various advantages and amplifies the impact of intermittent fasting.

THE BENEFITS OF INTERMITTENT FASTING

Fasting has been a fundamental practice in many cultures since ancient times. Still, its usage as a way of life and for health advantages, including weight reduction, is a relatively new phenomenon. Intermittent fasting as a healthy lifestyle choice has recently grown in popularity. The most important benefits of intermittent fasting are described below.

Aids in weight loss

Intermittent fasting, like any other kind of dieting, seeks to generate a calorie deficit, which means that the number of calories burnt is constantly higher than the number of calories consumed. When you fast for 16 hours or longer on a regular basis, your body becomes used to low-calorie intake and learns to utilize stored fat as fuel to supply energy for all physical activities.

If you continue to fast on a regular basis, you will lose inches from all of the areas of the body that are typically regarded as fat storage areas, such as the belly, hips, thighs, and so on. So, although weight reduction is not the primary goal of intermittent fasting, it is the practice's most essential and positive side effect since it increases the number of hormones that assist fat burning.

Avoids muscle loss

When you fast, your blood levels of human growth hormone (HGH) rise, increased hormone levels encourage fat burning to provide energy for the body, and once fat burning starts, it also aids in muscle growth. This, in turn, reduces muscle loss, which is typical in menopausal women.

Enhances metabolism

The fat-burning process starts with an increase in the levels of human growth hormone in the circulation, eventually leading to the body burning more calories to create the same amount of energy. This increases metabolic rate and aids in producing a calorie deficit between intake and outflow. Because you are fasting, your caloric intake is already decreased, and you burn more calories as your metabolic rate increases.

Reduces inflammation of cells

The human body is made up of endless cells that continue to develop until being destroyed and replaced by new cells at the end of their useful life. When continually eating, most of our body's energy and resources are dedicated toward food digestion. This leaves little or no time for the body to focus on cellular repair and rejuvenation.

There is a considerable gap between two eating sessions when we adopt the intermittent fasting diet. This time allows the body to repair damaged cells and prevents premature aging as well as illnesses such as cancer. However, when the cells are still functioning, they are subjected to wear and tear from regular physiological activities, which are typically restored while we sleep.

Enhances sleep quality

Improved sleep quality has been shown to reduce the aging process and reverse the effects of age. When an individual's general health improves, stress levels decrease, which leads to a decrease in cortisol levels, commonly known as the stress hormone. When stress is eliminated, getting a good night's sleep becomes much more manageable.

Better mental health

Intermittent fasting significantly reduces inflammation, anxiety, blood sugar, insulin resistance, and cholesterol and triglyceride levels. This results in fewer illnesses and disorders in the body. A healthy body is the home of a healthy mind. Depression and other diseases such as Alzheimer's keep away when the mind is healthy, bestowing the individual with excellent mental health.

Healthy/ balanced nutrition

Diet and lifestyle are the primary sources of health. You will likely be healthy if you feed your body the proper foods and live a healthy lifestyle. Short-term fasting may provide one health benefit over more regular meals. Fasting for brief periods of time activates autophagy, which is the breakdown of old or malfunctioning cells for use as fuel and the replacement of healthy cells.

Contributes to the overall improvement of health

Studies have shown that intermittent fasting has various health advantages, including lower cholesterol, triglycerides, blood sugar, and insulin resistance. The mind also relaxes when the body is calm, joyful, and healthy. A calm mind indicates lower cortisol levels as a consequence of less stress. Stress reduction leads to improved sleep, which leads to cellular repairs and the growth of organs in the body. All of this contributes to an increase in the individual's overall health. When our total health improves, we are able to live a longer, healthier life.

WHEN INTERMITTENT FASTING MAY BE INADVISABLE

Intermittent fasting is for everyone. Fasting is a way of life that is advocated and promoted in many ways across the globe by various religions, faiths, and sects. Fasting has been performed throughout the world from time immemorial. Nevertheless, certain persons are recommended against fasting. They are detailed below.

Pregnant Ladies and Lactating mothers

Pregnant women and breastfeeding moms, as is well known, supply nutrients to the fetus and baby. The new life needs sufficient nutrients to grow and develop, and it relies entirely on the mother for all its nutritional needs. If the mother begins fasting in this situation, she may lose out on sufficient nutrients and micronutrients that are essential for the newborn's healthy growth and development. As a result, pregnant women and breast-feeding moms are recommended to avoid intermittent fasting.

Individuals under the age of 18

Those under the age of 18 should avoid intermittent fasting and other types of dieting. This is because, while seeming to be fully grown adults, their bodies are still in the developing stage. Many physical and mental developing processes occur until the age of 18. This is the period when a well-balanced diet is critical for the individual's optimal growth and development. If these individuals turn to intermittent fasting at this time, they may miss out on development and may encounter various physical and mental concerns later in life.

Underweight individuals

Underweight people are already deficient in critical nutrients. They aren't receiving enough nutrients to keep their bodies running. They are at grave risk of being malnourished. As we all know, fasting causes the body to utilize stored fats and nutrients for energy. A body short in nutrition cannot offer the necessary lipids to burn for energy to keep the body operating. As a result, intermittent fasting is not recommended for underweight persons.

People suffering from eating disorders

Many individuals suffer from eating disorders such as anorexia, bulimia, and binge eating disorders. Such folks have a dysfunctional connection with eating.

They are either terrified of eating or consuming so much food that they are unable to manage their food intake. They subsequently over-exercise to punish themselves for overeating. Intermittent fasting is not advised for persons who have a negative relationship with eating. Fasting may do more damage than good for such folks.

People suffering from specific medical issues

Even if it causes insulin resistance, intermittent fasting is not recommended for patients with severe diabetes. This is due to the fact that intermittent fasting may alter your hormonal balance, insulin levels, and metabolism. Furthermore, people with diabetes are encouraged to eat something every couple of hours to regulate insulin levels and avoid hyperglycemia.

In such instances, it is highly advised to begin and maintain any fasting lifestyle in collaboration with and under the supervision of your doctor. People suffering from irritable bowel syndrome are in a similar situation. Fasting alters the way the digestive system operates. As a result, it is best to obtain professional advice before beginning any fast.

People suffering from mental illnesses

People with mental illnesses are often medicated heavily. Their bodies are already stressed from the medication's side effects, and their brains are anxious about their situation. Fasting, in addition to stress, induces hormonal changes, which may worsen the condition of such people. In such a case, mental problems would improve quicker if the body relieves the tension generated by fasting.

Athletes undergoing training

Training athletes come under the group of persons who need a lot of calories. When the body becomes used to intermittent fasting on a regular basis, the individual's total calorie intake decreases. This may have an impact on the athletes' training and energy levels. Though it is best avoided, athletes may practice intermittent fasting under the supervision of a competent dietitian or another skilled individual.

In conclusion, even though intermittent fasting has various health advantages, it should not be followed blindly. You should contact your doctor if you have certain pre-existing conditions or if you fall into the group of people who need a high-calorie intake for whatever reason.

A BEGINNER'S GUIDE

After learning about intermittent fasting in the preceding paragraphs, you may get the impression that it is a difficult practice. But don't worry, it's not complex. I've experienced the advantages of intermittent fasting and learned a lot.

The concepts of intermittent fasting outlined here are basic and straightforward to use in your daily life. All you need is some direction and information from my end, as well as some forethought on your side. I am eager to share all of my experiences, ideas, and techniques with you in order to assist you in restarting your weight reduction efforts and path to a healthy you.

Getting Started with Intermittent Fasting

It is as easy as breathing to begin an intermittent fast. However, transitioning into your new lifestyle requires some planning and preparation. I've compiled a list of points based on my intermittent fasting experiences to assist you in getting started on your intermittent fasting adventure.

Set your goal

Goal? Is it for fasting? Yes, a fasting aim. It would help if you weren't startled when I spoke about creating a plan before beginning intermittent fasting. This is because a trip cannot start unless a destination is determined.

This kind of excursion is known as wandering. If you are willing to fast occasionally, you should have a definite, attainable objective stated clearly and in solid character in a position immediately accessible to you. There is no way to know where you are going unless you have a goal in mind. The aim may be anything, such as dropping a few extra kilograms, improving one's health, lowering cholesterol or triglyceride levels, and so on.

Determine the best form of fasting for you

As previously said, there are several forms of intermittent fasting regimens. Examine each curriculum in depth to determine which one is ideal for you. Don't worry if your job prevents you from following the 16:8 fasting regimen.

There are no hard and fast rules that must be followed. You might follow the 5:2 diet, in which you usually eat throughout the week and fast on weekends with minimal calorie intake. Alternatively, you may eat for the first two days of the week, fast on the third, eat for two days again, and fast on the sixth. In that regard, intermittent fasting is a very adaptable approach.

You may fast whenever you want; consistency and discipline are only required. When you don't eat for 16 hours for a few days, your body adapts to the pattern and stops expecting meals during those 16 hours.

However, if you are inconsistent with your fasting or fasting periods, you will eat at random, generating tension and confusion in your internal functioning. You may begin or stop your fast an hour earlier or later than usual, but fasting for 16 hours on certain days and not fasting on others at will is not encouraged.

That is why you should first examine all of the fasting patterns available to you, as well as your daily routine, waking hours, work hours, and the time of day when you exercise, before deciding on the fasting pattern that is best for you.

Plan your fasting/eating schedule

You may wonder why it is necessary to plan for the eating time. You are free to eat anything you want. But that is not the case.

Missing major nutrients

When fasting for 16 hours a day, you must be highly conscious of what you consume during eating. This is because if you only eat for a few hours a day, you may lose out on essential macro and micronutrients needed for general bodily health if you do not organize your meals.

Meal proportions

You may also make the mistake of eating a substantial meal when you break the fast or a small meal before beginning your following fast. If this occurs, you will, for obvious reasons, lose out on the essence and advantages of fasting. Either be overly full during the eating period and miss the remaining meals, feeling hungry when it's time to fast, or you'll be hungry within a few hours of beginning your fast, making it tough to fast for the predetermined hours.

Incorporate it into your routine

Also, by the time you break the fast in the morning, you may have already been at your desk for a couple of hours. You won't be able to make anything and eat it for breakfast then, but if you had planned ahead of time, you'd have a nutritious, home-cooked meal ready to eat at your desk in no time.

Preparing meals ahead of time

When you plan your meals, you'll get an idea of what essential items you'll need to make those meals. You may also check for and acquire any missing materials ahead of time. Another significant advantage of meal planning is knowing in advance what nutrients you will be receiving from the food you will be consuming during that specific eating window.

With this information, you may balance out your meals if you find yourself overeating on any single dietary component. If you discover that a meal for a particular eating time is high in carbs, you may either modify some food items and add more protein-rich meals or balance it out the following day.

Fasting hours may be adjusted as needed.

Intermittent fasting is the most adaptable food and dieting strategy. If you choose a 16:8 fasting schedule and begin your fast at 7 pm, you may start your fast anytime between 6 and 8 pm.

BENEFITS BACKED UP BY SCIENCE

If it makes logical understanding, intermittent fasting can aid in weight loss. Food is broken down in our intestines by enzymes and ultimately ends up as particles in our circulation. Carbohydrates, especially sugars and refined grains (such as white flours and rice), are readily broken down into sugar, which our cells need for energy.

If our cells do not use it entirely, we store it as fat in our fat cells. However, sugar can only enter our cells with the help of insulin, which is a hormone made in the pancreas. Insulin delivers sugar into and retains it in fat cells.

As long as we don't snack during meals, our insulin levels will fall, allowing our fat cells to release their stored sugar for use as energy. We lose weight when we allow our insulin levels to fall. The whole point of intermittent fasting is to allow insulin levels to drop further and for long enough that we melt off our fat.

Some say that intermittent fasting is quite challenging. We do not think so. Here is why!

Human studies comparing fasting every other day versus eating less every day found that both worked roughly equally well for weight loss, albeit people have problems with the fasting days. So it's pretty reasonable to opt for a low-calorie plant-based, Mediterranean-style diet. However, evidence indicates that not all IF techniques are the same and that some IF diets are effective and sustainable, particularly when accompanied by a nutrient-rich diet.

We developed to be in rhythm with the cycle, known as a circadian rhythm. People usually eat during the day because it is known that daily food consumption is safe and does not lead to obesity. It has been said that obesity is highly linked with night eating.

Based on this, University of Alabama scientists ran a study with a tiny group of obese males with prediabetes. They contrasted "early time-restricted eating," a type of intermittent fasting in which all meals were packed into an early eight-hour interval of the day (7 am to 3 pm) or spaced out over 12 hours (between 7 am and 7 pm).

Both groups kept their weight (neither gained nor lost). Still, after five weeks, the first group had much lower insulin levels and insulin sensitivity and substantially lower blood pressure. The appetite was also dramatically reduced in the eight-hour group. What's the best part? They weren't going hungry.

Even participants who did not lose a single pound saw a significant improvement in metabolism simply by eating sooner in the day and prolonging the nighttime fast.

Why might shifting the timing be beneficial?

Fasting is deeply ingrained in our physiology, activating several critical cellular activities. But what impact does simply shifting the timing have to do with fasting and our bodies? A comprehensive review of the science of IF published recently in the New England Journal of Medicine gives some light.

Switching from a diet to a fast state does more than just help us burn fat and lose weight. The research teams scoured through large numbers of animal and human studies to clarify how simple fasting enhances metabolism decreases blood sugar levels, and reduces inflammation. Fasting decreases various health issues ranging from conditions such as arthritis to asthma and even aids in the removal of toxins and damaged cells, which reduces the risk of cancer and strengthens brain function.

Is intermittent fasting as beneficial as it sounds?

"There is evidence suggesting that the fasting method, where meals are constrained to an eight to ten-hour daytime period, is effective," says metabolic specialist Dr. Deborah Wexler. Nonetheless, she advises people to "adopt an eating method that ensures for them and is affordable to them."

So, here's the situation. There is some excellent scientific evidence that, when eaten in moderation and lifestyle, fasting has the power to be a particularly successful method of weight loss, particularly for persons at risk of diabetes. (However, those with advanced diabetes or on diabetes medications, people with a history of eating disorders such as anorexia and bulimia, and those that are pregnant or breastfeeding should not engage in it.

Four ways to apply this knowledge to improve your health.

- Sugar and refined cereals should be avoided. Consume fruits and vegetables, beans and lentils, whole grains, lean meats, and healthy fat alternatives.
- Increase muscle tone. Allow your body to burn fat in between meals. Keep moving throughout the day.
- Consider a basic example of intermittent fasting. Restrict the hours you consume food, and eat earlier in the day for the best results.
- Always avoid snacking as well as eating late at night.

We have finished this chapter with the four scientifically approved ways in which intermittent fasting can be beneficial. In the next chapter, learn how intermittent fasting can benefit your health as an over-50 woman and how it can be your ticket to keeping a healthy weight throughout your golden years.

SELF-ASSESSMENT TEST:

1. What have you learned in this chapter?

2. Based on everything that you have learned, consider your unique circumstances and then make the following lists:

   a) Reasons why you think intermittent fasting may be suitable for you.

   b) Reasons why you believe intermittent fasting may not be ideal for you.

3

OKAY, BUT IS IT SAFE AND EFFECTIVE FOR WOMEN OVER 50?

Weight increase in women over the age of 40 is relatively prevalent, while the specific reason and effect are still being debated. Lower estrogen levels may indicate a slower metabolic rate, which can lead to weight gain even if our diet remains unchanged.

Because of increasing insulin resistance, we may be less able to metabolize carbs and sugars. Or it could be that the two fat-storing enzymes, which are much more effective in postmenopausal women, are contributing to menopause weight increase. Or it could be that muscle mass loss causes us to burn fewer calories while resting. Unfortunately, many women have an increase in ghrelin, also known as the hunger hormone, and/or a reduction in leptin, the hormone that signals when we're full.

One of the first things to grasp is that gaining weight at this age (or any age) is not a sign of "failure" or a lack of willpower. Beating yourself up about it isn't only inaccurate, but it also doesn't burn calories, so don't do it. Hormones have far more influence on our actions and emotions, and swings in estrogen levels, right after a drop in estrogen levels, can make weight control much more difficult.

One of the most significant and most up-to-date evaluations of the studies on intermittent fasting in adult women, published in JAMA Network Open, found that intermittent fasting indeed helps with moderate weight loss, with proof ranging from medium to high quality.

To obtain this result, the researchers examined 11 published meta-analyses combined with looking at 130 different randomized controlled trials. Further investigation revealed that only the 5:2 or a comparable adjusted alternate-day fast was related to "a statistically meaningful weight loss of more than 5% in people with overweight or obesity." They discovered that time-restricted eating, such as the Galveston diet, did not provide equivalent results.

Furthermore, the researchers highlight that IF appeared to be most effective in the first between one to six months, after which participants frequently encountered a weight plateau.

Women, it is true, are the captives of their hormones. A woman's body constantly changes throughout her life, from childhood to adolescence, through menstruation, pregnancy, perimenopause, menopause, and finally, postmenopause. Aside from the physical changes that occur, many hormonal changes mark the beginning of each phase of a woman's life.

The quantity of estrogen, the female hormone secreted in the body, plays a critical role at each stage. All of the dynamic changes significantly impact the woman's thinking, affecting her self-image and positivity.

MENOPAUSE JUST MAKES THINGS WORSE

Menopause is the final stage of the menstrual cycle. Women have reached the end of their reproductive years. Menopause is said to begin when a woman goes 12 months without menstruating. Menopause often occurs between the ages of 45 and 55, depending on the woman's ethnicity, genetics, and family history. It is a normal part of the aging process.

Menopause is the typical reduction of reproductive hormones that occurs when a woman reaches her late 40s or early 50s. This is a case of "sudden" or "premature" menopause. Menopause could also occur surgically when a woman's ovaries are surgically removed.

What causes menopause?

The menstrual cycle, which begins in adolescence, decreases and eventually ends as you age. Ovaries are crucial reproductive organs because they store eggs and discharge them into the fallopian tubes. They also manufacture estrogen, progesterone, and testosterone. As menopause approaches, the ovaries produce less estrogen.

Estrogen with progesterone works together to regulate the menstrual cycle. So, as estrogen levels drop, it disrupts your menstrual cycle, causing irregular menstruation at first and ultimately stopping completely.

Estrogen levels affect a woman's biology more than just menstrual management. Estrogen is in charge of calcium utilization in a woman's body and regulates cholesterol levels. As the body adjusts to the lower estrogen levels, it undergoes a number of changes. These are the symptoms associated with the beginning of menopause.

Stages of Menopause

Menopause does not happen all at once. It is a lengthy process that involves a succession of changes in a woman's body over a period of 5 to 15 years. Menopause is further classified into three stages, which are as follows:

Perimenopause - Perimenopause begins in the late thirties or early forties. It is the time when the ovaries begin to decrease estrogen production. This time often begins 8-10 years before the beginning of menopause. Menopause symptoms appear in the last 1-2 years of perimenopause.

Menopause - Menopause occurs when the ovaries stop producing eggs and menstruation ceases altogether. It usually happens due to low hormone levels, and it starts somewhere between 45 years and 55 years old. There are cases in which it happens earlier.

Post menopause - The period immediately following menopause when the body adjusts to a lower amount of estrogen and the lack of the monthly cycle is known as postmenopause. The majority of menopausal symptoms occur during this time. Furthermore, women are more susceptible to osteoporosis or heart disease at this time, and the risk of disorders associated with estrogen deficiency grows with age.

Menopause symptoms

Every woman is different; her menstrual cycles are distinctive, as is her menopausal experience. It is not necessary for what one woman goes through throughout menopause to be shared by other women.

The following are the most often observed symptoms:

- Flashes of heat
- Weight increase around the abdomen
- Vaginal dryness
- Insomnia
- If not handled promptly, emotional changes might develop into depression.
- Swings in mood
- Skin, eyes, and mouth that are dry
- Fatigue
- Headaches
- Aches and pains in the joints and muscles
- Loss of hair
- Libido deficiency

Premature menopause

Your genes, immune system issues, or surgical procedures can all induce premature menopause. Endometriosis and uterine cancer require surgical treatments to be treated. Ovaries can potentially be damaged by radiation or chemotherapy.

Menopause treatment

Menopause is a normal process that occurs in women as they get older. It isn't an illness that requires treatment. Specific symptoms manifest themselves more prominently in some women than in others.

Medical attention

Most symptoms will go away with time, but if you feel that they are interfering with your life in any way, you should visit your doctor.

Following a review of your situation, the doctor may propose a course of action, including hormone replacement therapy (HRT), non-hormone therapy, and/or osteoporosis drugs. It is essential to highlight that HRT has numerous adverse effects and should only be used as a last resort.

INTERMITTENT FASTING - THE ESSENTIAL AID REGARDING MENOPAUSE

We discussed the indications and symptoms of menopause in the preceding paragraphs. Making certain lifestyle adjustments is one crucial line of treatment indicated for menopausal symptoms. Adjusting to intermittent fasting is one such lifestyle shift. Intermittent fasting alleviates some key menopausal symptoms by doing the following:

Weight control

Slowly and steadily breaking down fat to create energy aids in weight loss. Intermittent fasting, as outlined in previous chapters, aids in creating a calorie deficit by cycling between eating and fasting periods. Longer fasting durations result in the usage of body fat, a process known as ketosis, to provide energy for bodily activities—this aids in the utilization of the body's fat reserves. Thus, intermittent fasting aids in female weight management.

Enhances sleep quality

Intermittent fasting aids in the reinforcement of your circadian rhythms. Circadian rhythm is the body's biological clock or internal clock that governs all bodily functions.

When mealtimes are managed, the body instinctively adjusts the sleep cycle to match. This improves sleep quality and allows you to get deep, effortless sleep.

Enhances metabolism

Intermittent fasting improves metabolism, as explained in the following chapter. It controls calorie intake, leading to a deficit between actual calorie requirements and calorie intake, leading to weight loss and enhanced metabolism.

Inflammation, aches, and pains are reduced.

Menopause is characterized by inflammation in many body sections and aches and pains in the joints and muscles. Intermittent fasting's extended fasting intervals allow the body to repair and regenerate cells, lowering inflammation at the cellular level. If done correctly, intermittent fasting can even aid with conditions like cancer and Alzheimer's.

Diabetes risk is reduced, and heart health is improved.

The more extended fasting periods of intermittent fasting aid in lowering blood insulin levels. When you fast for a more extended period of time, your body does not receive a fresh supply of carbs to convert the glucose from it into fuel to generate energy. In the long run, this lowers insulin levels as well as triglyceride and cholesterol levels. In menopausal women, intermittent fasting reduces the risk of diabetes and improves heart health. The decrease in estrogen levels that occurs with the onset of menopause impacts heart health and may lead to insulin resistance and diabetes.

PSYCHOLOGICAL ADVANTAGES

- Increased Concentration: From an evolutionary standpoint, it is possible to believe that certain cognitive functions are weakened after eating. This is to be expected because, after eating, the sympathetic nervous system, which is required to initiate cognitive tasks, is muted, and the parasympathetic nervous system is engaged. Furthermore, research shows that fasting increases the neurotransmitters involved with the psychological state of concentration, like norepinephrine and orexin.
- Neuroplasticity, or the brain's ability to form new connections, is improved: Entering ketosis and rotating among different energy sources enhances brain plasticity.
- Antidepressant properties. BDNF (brain-derived neurotrophic factor), a chemical produced by the brain, is nearly non-existent in sad persons. Increasing its production protects against depression. Intermittent fasting can help with this.
- Reading speed while learning.
- Prevention of inflammatory processes
- Inflammatory processes can conflict with nervous system function. When confronted

with this state, the body directs its resources toward fighting inflammation while reducing cognitive capabilities. So, by reducing inflammation in the body through fasting times, we urge those resources to be devoted to what is necessary.

- Food seeking reduction: It assists us in recognizing hunger and satiety signals, supporting us in avoiding emotional or dull hunger.
- The way we consume, mainly if ultra-processed foods are included in our diet, causes insulin spikes that cause mental weariness. These peaks are lowered if we eat natural and "good processed" foods after fasting. Mental fatigue is reduced.

In short, intermittent fasting has numerous advantages, including a reduction in symptoms and discomfort associated with the onset of menopause in women.

Let's not forget that people are also confused because there is no agreement on what constitutes a healthy diet. Is there a low-fat diet that they should follow? Are you sick of carbs? Under-calorie? Do you like sugar? Do you have a low glycemic index? It is easier to understand with a fundamentally different fasting strategy. It can be described in just a few words: Nothing to do but sleep.

That's all! Diets might fail due to ineffectiveness and lack of sufficient follow-up. Fasting's most evident benefit is its simplicity, which is also the primary reason for its success. When it comes to dietary laws, the simpler, the better.

Of course, in a perfect world, everyone would eat organic veggies and grass-fed cattle instead of white bread or overly processed foods. The fact remains that organic foods can cost up to ten times as much as industrial commodities.

Cereals are subsidized by the government, making them significantly more affordable than other foods. As a result, 2 pounds of cherries can cost $8 or $9, yet a baguette is worth approximately $1, and a packet of pasta is worth much less. It is considerably easier to feed a family on a low budget with pasta and white bread.

Cooking requires time, for sure. Purchasing, preparing the food, cooking time, and cleaning time. Everything takes time, and time is a precious commodity that is often in short supply. Even with the greatest of inten-tions, instructing everyone to cook isn't the best technique if you want to see results. Fasting requires additional shopping, preparation supplies, cooking, and cleanup. It's a method of making your life easier. Fasting is a convenient practice. There is nothing to do. Many schemes include instructions. Nothing is required for fasting. It's challenging to keep things simple!

Many diets advise making the ice cream or dessert a precise cross. That is excellent weight-loss advice. However, putting it into action is difficult. It goes on to say to abstain for six months or even a year, but what about the rest of your days? And why would you want to? Consider that for a moment. What could be more fun than assembling the piece and toasting with a bottle of champagne at your best friend's wedding?

Do you want to give up those delights for good? Why not make a birthday salad instead of a birthday cake? Isn't it true that existence has lost some of its lusters? There is plenty of time to live. Fasting after sprains can help restore balance. That is the essence of the life cycle. Drought is followed by abundance.

Overflowing is caused by starvation. It has always been like that. Birthdays, weddings, parties, and other special occasions have traditionally been associated with feasts since time immemorial. Such feasts, however, must be followed by fasts. You can tolerate aberrations by not eating until you correct them. Fasting is, above all, about achieving homeostasis.

Many persons with type 2 diabetes are overweight and have significant insulin resistance. Even a rigorous ketogenic diet (minimal carbohydrates, moderate protein, and plenty of fat) is sometimes insufficient to combat the illness.

In those conditions, fasting is the simplest and most effective strategy to reduce insulin and improve insulin resistance. Fasting is effective for overcoming the stages of weight loss and decreasing insulin requirements.

The key therapeutic benefit is that the number of fasts that can be done is not limited. The longest known fast lasted 382 days and had no adverse effects on the sufferer. If the fast does not produce the desired results, simply increase the frequency or length until the desired outcome is obtained. Diets that are low in fat, low in carbohydrates (low carb), or paleo-style work for some people but not for others. If you don't see any diet results, you won't have much room to improve it.

Fasting, however, requires just that you extend the time! The faster you move, the more probable it is that you will lose weight, although this will always occur.

Many diets involve eating first thing in the morning and then splitting meals for the remainder of the day every two and a half hours. That type of diet works nicely for certain folks. Nonetheless, obtaining and preparing food six, seven, or eight times per day is incredibly tough.

There is no specified time limit. However, you can travel for 16 hours or 16 days at any time. You can fast one day every week, five days the following week, and two days the next week. Fasting adjusts to your duties and allows you to combine multiple durations without being trapped in a routine.

The latest magic weapon for healthy and permanent weight loss is intermittent fasting, which involves not eating for 16 hours. Aside from that, intermittent fasting should reduce inflammation in the body and lower blood pressure. Is it a fad or a sensible source of nutrition? Here are the facts.

In a nutshell, intermittent fasting is the practice of not eating for 16 hours, saving for water, unsweetened teas, and black coffee. Drinking a lot is even required. For the next 8 hours, you can eat normally. There are no limitations. It is also up to you whether you forego breakfast or (late) dinner.

When you ingest something, it is subdivided into its constituents and released into your bloodstream. Your blood sugar level will rise if you consume carbohydrates. In order to control this, your body produces more insulin to transfer sugar molecules from the blood to the cells that require them (e.g., brain, heart, muscles). Your cells prefer to use sugar for energy as long as blood sugar and insulin levels are elevated. Fat burning is therefore reduced to a bare minimum.

Your blood sugar and insulin levels stay consistent when you don't eat, and your body depends more on existing fat deposits. This boosts fat metabolism and soothes the digestive system. Other benefits include: Interval fasting has been shown to reduce inflammation, regulate blood pressure, and encourage the growth of new brain cells. It is, by the way, not a new "innovation." When people had to hunt and gather their food, they were accustomed to long meal breaks, which the body "optimized" for.

A negative energy balance is required. In other words, you must expend more energy than you consume. So, consume balanced and healthful food during your eating periods, and add regular exercise into your daily routine. You don't want to skip your morning workout, but your first meal of the day is only "allowed" at noon.

In addition, intermittent fasting can help you lose weight sustainably and non-yo-yo.

That is not an issue. Training on an empty stomach, on the other hand, provides advantages. Your training will be more successful if you focus on your stress areas. However, it would be best if you worked out in the area of fat metabolism. If you are always on the go, the energy from fat burning will not suffice. Because carbohydrates are unavailable, your body relies on muscle protein. This has a long-term negative impact on muscle mass, lowers performance, and weakens your immune system.

WHAT IS THE BEST INTERMITTENT FASTING ROUTINE?

There are none. Arrange your non-meal hours in the manner that is most convenient for you. The 16/8 form can also be altered. This is the most prevalent, but other possibilities are 18/6 or 20/4. Another option is to alternate between fasting days and "regular feeding days." Or you can wager on "5-to-2" and fast two days a week while eating normally the other five. But more on that in the next chapter. Let's wrap this up now.

Because intermittent fasting is not a diet but rather a form of eating regimen, it is permanent. It is critical that you feel good and that you can easily incorporate your diet into your daily life. Suppose intermittent fasting causes you compulsion and stress. In that case, it makes no sense and will have the opposite impact regarding weight loss because "stress hormones" encourage sugar consumption while inhibiting fat burning. In the following chapter, we'll examine the many types of intermittent fasting.

4

TYPES OF INTERMITTENT FASTING—WHICH ONE SHOULD YOU FOLLOW?

You may believe that fasting is fasting, fasting, and more fasting. No, not at all. Fasting is abstaining from calorie-containing foods and liquids, although there are other approaches. As intermittent fasting has grown in popularity, it has branched out into different varieties to accommodate the expanding number of people with varying needs and tastes.

Some methods of intermittent fasting are more effective for some people than others. Some are easier to follow and maintain statistically than others. Let's examine the many intermittent fasting programs available to decide which is best for you.

- Intermittent fasting programs come in a variety of forms, including:
- The intermittent fasting plan of 16:8
- The 5:2 intermittent fasting plan
- The Fast 800 Program
- Choose Your Intermittent Fasting Day
- Warrior Diet Intermittent fasting (Eat Stop Eat)
- Intermittent fasting on alternate days

We'll review each in terms of popularity, success rate, and female suitability.

16:8 INTERMITTENT FASTING IS THE MOST POPULAR ONE

The 16:8 intermittent fasting is also known as the 16:8 plan or the 16:8 diet. It is also known as the Leangains approach, time-restricted fasting (TMF), time-restricted eating (TME), or time-restricted feeding (TMF). The name says it all; you fast for 16 hours per day and have an eight-hour window to eat your allotted calories. This is now one of the most popular intermittent fasting regimens accessible, and many people find it the easiest to keep to over time.

How do you do this one?

You can pretty much plan your intermittent fasting plan around your daily schedule. However, scheduling your eight-hour eating window within the day's middle hours is usually ideal. Why in the middle of the day? It is thought that eating in the middle of the day best complements the normal human circadian cycle.

In other words, it closely resembles eating times set by your natural internal clock. Diurnal and crepuscular creatures are the two sorts of animals that are awake during the day. Crepuscular creatures are most active around twilight and morning and rest during the day. Diurnal animals are active throughout the day and feed in the middle of the day. While some people like to stay awake at night and maybe be branded as "night owls," humans are essentially diurnal.

This places the 16:8 intermittent fasting eating window right in the middle of your natural pattern. Another advantage of the 16:8 diet is that you may manage your eating window such that your last meal is at a decent time before bed. This is likely one of the reasons why this intermittent fasting diet is so simple to follow.

What is the significance of this? It has been proposed that waiting for two to four hours between your last meal and retiring to bed may have health benefits.

During this time, your meal is partially digested as it moves from your stomach to your intestines.

One advantage is that it minimizes potential heartburn and reflux when you lie down. You are also not putting your body into 'idle mode with a full stomach, which naturally slows down all physical functions, including digestion and metabolism. Eating too close to bedtime may also interfere with your sleep quality. The release of insulin by your body is linked to your internal clock. When insulin is released after a meal, your body may get agitated.

Trying to relax before bed can cause difficulty falling and staying asleep, preventing you from getting a decent night's sleep. Another devious twist is up the 16:8 intermittent fasting plan's sleeve. Adults usually require seven to nine hours of sleep per night. When you set your 16:8 eating window in the middle of the day, you intend to sleep for seven to nine hours of your fasting time. This means you spend less time experiencing the negative symptoms of fasting, such as hunger.

Variation and adaptability

The option of modification and flexibility is an appealing element of the usual 16:8 intermittent fasting diet. You are not restricted to specific times to begin and end your fast. You can start and finish whenever you choose. Even if you work a shift, you can change your fasting period to fit your waking and sleeping hours. You also do not need to follow a strict 16:8 diet. You can experiment with different fasting periods to see what works best for you. Among the variations are:

- 12:12
- 14:10
- 16:8
- 18:6
- 20:4

You can extend or shorten your fasting period based on how long you can go without eating. As you get used to the intermittent fasting lifestyle, you can start with a smaller fasting window and progressively extend it. For example, you may begin with the 12:12 version for a week or two, then go to the 14:10, and so on until you find the fasting-eating ratio that works best for you.

Women starting the 16:8 intermittent fasting regimen should aim for a shorter fasting period of 14 to 15 hours at a time. This is because women appear to perform better with shorter fasting periods in which they refrain entirely from food.

Scheduled meal times include:

- 9:00 a.m. to 5:00 p.m.
- 10:00 a.m. to 6:00 p.m.
- 12 pm to 8:00 pm.

It would be best to plan your eating window around your regular schedule. For instance, if you don't get home until 6 pm, eat dinner at approximately 7 pm, and go to bed around 10 pm, your eating window must be between 11 am and 7 pm. This allows you to sleep two to three hours after your last meal and corresponds to your normal waking and active hours.

WOMEN'S FAVOURITE: INTERMITTENT FASTING 5:2

The fast diet is another name for the 5:2 intermittent fasting strategy. It's popular and a great place to start for anyone who wants to attempt intermittent fasting but is put off by more extreme fasting programs. This is arguably the most simple intermittent fasting plan available. It allows you to "dip your toes in the water," so to speak, without committing to long periods of no meals or even entire days.

The 5:2 regimen is also regarded as women's most effective intermittent fasting schedule. Shorter fasting times benefit women more than more extended fasting periods. Fasting can affect your hormones as a woman, affecting fertility and causing an imbalance. Hence shorter fasts are preferable. The 5:2 fasting strategy reduces the stress on your body and, as a result, the impact on your hormones. So, how exactly does the 5:2 plan work?

How do you do it?

The 5:2 intermittent fasting regimen is divided into two parts. You usually eat five days per week. You follow an extremely low-calorie diet two days a week. What's that? Where is the fasting in this? There is no extreme fasting with the 5:2 regimen, which contributes to its ease of implementation and makes it an excellent stepping stone for easing into intermittent fasting. Once you've mastered this strategy, you might want to take it a step further and practice a stricter kind of intermittent fasting that entails complete abstinence from food.

Another aspect of this plan's popularity is its flexibility. You can choose which days to arrange as 'fasting' days and which to eat normally from week to week. The sole scheduling constraint is having at least one non-fasting day between your two fasting days. With such a high degree of adaptability, you can personalize your fasting schedule to your specific needs. For example, if your life focuses on routine plus planning, you can keep the same fasting days every week. If your life is more casual or if you have no established routine, you can pick and choose your fasting days as you go.

Another advantage of the 5:2 plan's adaptability is that you don't have to feel awkward in social situations because you're the only one who isn't eating or drinking. People who follow intermittent fasting frequently shun social events, especially in the beginning. If you have an event to attend on a designated fasting day—a birthday, a girls' night out, etc.—you can simply plan your fasting day for the day before or after.

Remember to not double-stack your fasting days and to leave at least one 'regular' day in between. You can have your cake and eat it too by maintaining your social life while also practicing intermittent fasting. We previously stated that the 5:2 diet does not include any genuine fasting in which you abstain from food for an extended period of time. So, how exactly does this work? On fasting days, you limit your daily caloric intake to 500 calories. You can choose to consume two tiny meals of 250 calories each, or you can graze on very low-calorie foods throughout the day, such as small salads. It is entirely up to you how you fill those 500 calories.

It is critical that you consume a regular, healthy diet on non-fasting days. Binge on junk food can raise your calorie intake and negate the benefits of fasting. Worse, it may result in weight gain. Maintain a balanced diet that supplies you with all of the nourishment you require while not exceeding your specific daily calorie needs.

THE FAST 800 PROGRAM

The Fast 800 is a staggering intermittent fasting technique developed by Dr. Michael Mosley. It involves no challenging fasting, hence no complete abstinence from meals, like the classic 5:2 intermittent fasting diet. It consists of three distinct stages:

- The Extremely Fast 800
- The New 5:2 Lifestyle
- The Very Fast 800

The plan's initial stage is designed for rapid weight loss and should be followed for at least two weeks. The length of time you stay in the first stage will be determined by your level of comfort as well as your weight loss goals. If you believe you can keep up with the plan's first stage, you can do so for a total of 12 weeks or three months.

You eat only 800 calories daily, every day, during this program stage. Adopting a Mediterranean diet is perfect for this type of low-calorie diet since it fills you up on nutritious foods that keep you feeling fuller for longer.

However, this aggressive strategy for weight loss based on a low-calorie diet for two to twelve weeks is not for everyone. Compared to the 5:2 technique discussed above, it can be hard to maintain a low-calorie diet for longer. The New 5:2 diet is the name of the second stage of this regimen. This stage is based on the standard 5:2 intermittent fasting diet. You will choose two days per week to 'fast.'

For the remaining five days of the week, you will eat regularly. This stage of the plan provides the same level of freedom as the 5:2 diet. You get to choose which days to fast, and you can alter them from week to week, as long as you have at least one free day between your two fasting days. This program's second stage can be continued indefinitely or until your health and weight loss goals are accomplished.

When you determine you no longer wish to fast, you can progress to the program's Way of Life stage. The third level of the program is a maintenance plan called Way of Life, named because it simply involves the act of continuing to eat a healthy, balanced diet.

Maintaining your progress once you've achieved your goals is critical; otherwise, you'll have to start all over again. Some people may benefit significantly from a staggering method to an intermittent fasting regimen. Instead of merely getting off the intermittent fasting bus, it begins more aggressively and concludes in maintenance. It may also be simpler to stick to than other intermittent fasting strategies, including challenging periods where you don't eat anything for extended periods.

CHOOSE YOUR INTERMITTENT FASTING DAY

This intermittent fasting strategy is similar to the 16:8 Intermittent Fasting method, but with a twist. It is similar to the intermittent fasting strategy of "skipping a meal every other day."

Instead of fasting for a certain period of time every day, you do it every other day or a few times a week. You can fast in the same manner as the 16:8 approach or modify your fasting period depending on your mood and inclination.

Remember that women respond better to shorter fasting periods, so it's usually ideal to fast for 14 hours at a time rather than longer. If you think you can handle it for a little longer on a specific day, go for it. If you think you won't be able to fast on a particular day, that's fine; don't. This is especially effective if you are sick and believe fasting will make you feel worse.

As an example:

- Monday – Eat as usual.
- Tuesday – Eat as usual.
- Wednesday - Fast from Tuesday night's dinner till noon on Wednesday.
- Thursday – Eat as usual.
- Friday — Fast from Thursday night's dinner till mid-afternoon on Friday.
- Saturday – Eat as usual.
- Sunday - Fast from Saturday night's dinner to late Sunday morning.

The objective is to fast a couple of times a week for 12 to 14 hours or longer without having to stick to this scheduled day in and day out, day after day.

WARRIOR DIET INTERMITTENT FASTING (EAT STOP EAT)

Ori Hofmekler developed the Warrior Diet in 2001. The regimen is based on the eating habits of ancient warriors. They would not eat much during the day but would feast at night. It's worth noting that Hofmekler himself confesses that this diet isn't solely based on research. It is also based on his personal thoughts and observations of people who have followed this diet while serving in the Israeli Special Forces.

This is yet another intermittent fasting diet program that does not require prolonged food deprivation. It focuses on what is known as undereating. You can eat, but the meals you eat during your fast must be incredibly low-calorie or zero calories items.

How do you do it?

The Warrior Diet follows a 20:4 fasting to eating ratio, in which you fast or restrict calories for 20 hours of the day and feast for four hours—consuming limited amounts of low-calorie vegetables, fruits, and some dairy and eggs are suggested throughout the fasting period. Drinking plenty of zero-calorie drinks is essential, as it is with other intermittent fasting diets.

After your 20-hour fasting phase is over, you can eat whatever you want to make up your daily calories. Nevertheless, there is a caveat to this story: Going wild does not mean surpassing your daily caloric demands, as this will result in weight increase rather than weight loss.

During the 20-hour fasting phase, you should not ingest more than 10% to 15% of your daily calorie needs. You should consume 85 to 90 percent of your daily caloric demands throughout your four-hour fasting window. While feasting may result in overeating if you binge on junk food, if you follow a balanced diet, you are likely to consume fewer calories than you require. This generates a calorie deficit, which, paired with not eating for the other 20 hours of the day, may result in rapid weight reduction.

For most people, this is not a viable intermittent fasting plan. This diet causes many problems and can have hazardous side effects. This cycle of restricting calories and bingeing might quickly evolve to bulimic disordered eating, which could have long-term negative consequences.

Another disadvantage of the Warrior Diet is the very real risk of malnutrition. Receiving all the required nutrients might be challenging when you eat only one main meal daily. To ensure that you obtain the nourishment your body needs, it is recommended that you consume a healthy, balanced diet rich in a variety of nutrient-dense foods.

The Warrior Diet, like the Fast 800 diet, can be condensed down into a three-week regimen to get you started. After the first three weeks, you can decide how and if you want to continue based on your health and weight loss goals. After completing the initial three-week presentation, Hofmekler advises either cycling through the phases from the start or actively pushing with the third stage until your goals are met.

Week one, often known as phase one: During the 20-hour fast, consume tiny amounts of low-calorie fruits, vegetables, vegetable juices, dairy, eggs, or clear broth. Consume a salad with vinegar plus oil dressing and one or more large meals consisting of non-wheat whole grains, plant proteins, some cooked vegetables, and dairy products such as cheese. Drink plenty of zero-calorie beverages throughout the day, such as water, coffee, tea, and a little milk. The goal is to consume only 15% of your daily caloric requirements.

Week two, or phase two, of the diet is a high-fat period. During the 20-hour fast, consume tiny amounts of low-calorie fruits, vegetables, vegetable juices, dairy, eggs, or clear broth. The goal is to consume only 15% of your daily caloric requirements. Consume a salad with vinegar, oil dressing, and one or more large meals consisting of cooked lots of veggies, animal protein, and a minimum of one, preferably two, handfuls of nuts. During this phase, all starches and grains are removed.

Week three, often known as phase three: For your feasting period, the third step of the diet plan rotates between high-protein days and high-carb days. You

adhere to the same 20-hour under-eating recommen-
dations as in phases one and two but alternate between
high protein and high carb days at night. For example,
one or two days of heavy carbohydrate and moderate
protein consumption. One to two days of rich protein
and minimal carbs. One or two days of heavy carbohydrate and moderate protein consumption. And so forth.

EAT STOP EAT

At first look, the Eat Stop Eat approach appears to be
similar to the Alternate Day intermittent fasting
method. However, they are not. Fasting is practiced
twice a week when following the Eat Stop Eat
approach. Your fasting days are separated by two non-
fasting days. While this spacing results in two fasting
days per week, there will be a week with three fasting
days in seven days. As an example:

- Monday – Eat as usual.
- Tuesday – Eat as usual.
- Wednesday is a fast day.
- Thursday – Eat as usual.
- Friday - Eat as usual.
- Saturday is a fast day.
- Sunday – Eat as usual.

However, every now and then, you'll have a week like this:

- Monday is a fast day.
- Tuesday – Eat as usual.
- Wednesday – Eat as usual.
- Thursday is a fast day.
- Friday - Eat as usual.
- Saturday – Eat as usual.
- Sunday is a fast day.

The Eat Stop Eat intermittent fasting strategy is precisely that. You eat normally for two days, then go on a 24-hour or whole-day fast. During this fast, you can only drink zero-calorie liquids like unsweetened coffee and tea with no added milk, cream, or creamer, as well as water or zero-sugar carbonated drinks.

For instance, if you have dinner at 6:00 pm on Monday, your fast will extend until 6:00 pm on Tuesday, when you will eat again. You will then eat your proper meals until Thursday night before restarting your fast after supper on Thursday night and fasting until dinner on Friday night.

You can choose which meal is your last; dinner may be a good option because you will spend the first portion of your 24-hour fast asleep, limiting the amount of time you feel hungry throughout those 24 hours. If you have breakfast as your last meal, you will merely sleep through the latter portion of your 24-hour fast, making you feel hungry sooner rather than later.

Consume a nutritious, balanced diet and keep track of how much you eat on non-fasting days to avoid compensating for the lost calories. On 'regular' days, you may overeat without even realizing it. While fasting will burn fat on fasting days, if you overeat on non-fasting days, you will put it all back on just as quickly as you are burning it.

INTERMITTENT FASTING ON ALTERNATE DAYS

Fasting on alternate days is also known as 1:1 intermittent fasting. Many people find it challenging to keep to this strategy of intermittent fasting. You eat regularly every other day and fast on the other. This fasting strategy does not involve long periods of total abstinence from meals.

Instead, during fasting days, you reduce your calorie intake. Personal choice determines what you wish to limit your calories too. You can get ideas for your fasting day calorie limit from either the classic 5:2 diet or the Fast 800 Diet. In general, you should limit your-self to 500 to 800 calories per day.

If you decide to try Alternate Day Fasting and start with a 500-calorie limit but find it challenging to stick to, consider increasing your calories to 800. Once your body adjusts to the alternating fasting regimen, you can always reduce it back to 500.

As with the Eat Stop Eat approach, eat a healthy, balanced diet and keep track of how much you eat on non-fasting days to avoid compensating for the missed calories. While fasting will burn fat on fasting days, if you overeat on non-fasting days, you will put it back on just as quickly as you are burning it. On 'regular' days, you may overeat without even realizing it.

We are all aware that intermittent fasting is the most basic of diets with health benefits for those who follow it. However, some guidelines for the dos and don'ts of intermittent fasting are discussed below.

WHAT YOU SHOULD DO

Consult with your doctor.

Several studies have demonstrated that intermittent fasting benefits individuals who practice it. Humans have followed it from the beginning of time. When there was no electricity, early humans ate their last meal of the day before nightfall, and their next meal was only after daybreak the next day.

Intermittent fasting has grown in favor of a way of life and nutrition in recent years. This resulted in a regular fast of more than 14 hours. And while it has numerous advantages, like with any other diet or fitness plan, it is best to consult your doctor before embarking on your fasting journey.

This is due to the fact that your doctor and dietitian are the ideal individuals to advise you on what is best for you based on your pre-existing health conditions, age, and lifestyle. They are the experts who can point out the benefits and drawbacks of any diet for you as a person because what works for one person may not work for the next.

Plan your meals ahead of time.

In intermittent fasting, the eating window is your body's 'building' phase. As the fasting or 'elimination' phase has helped your body get rid of the dead and disease-causing cells and other accumulated toxins, all of your body's cells are like sponges. The body is ready to take all of its nutrients to form new cells, muscles, and neurons.

Now, suppose you organize your meals to include all the key food components, such as proteins, carbs, fats, fibers, vitamins, minerals, and other micronutrients. In that case, you will offer your body with all of the raw materials it requires to give you the gift of good health and mental serenity. As a result, it is critical to schedule your meals ahead of time so that when mealtime arrives, you may eat good and wholesome food and get the full benefits of fasting.

Make sure to include all food varieties.

Many experts feel that when following the intermittent fasting pattern or lifestyle, you should avoid dieting during the eating window between fasts and eat a variety of foods. This is because when you are fasting, your body does not receive a new supply of carbs to convert into energy. During these periods, the body summonsed the fat stored in cells to be broken down and converted into energy for the body's functions.

Furthermore, your food intake is significantly reduced because you are fasting for most of the day. Moreover, you may fail to include certain vital nutrients in your meals, which may lead to malnutrition in the long run.

Exercise!

Exercise is the most important aspect of any lifestyle modification. Exercise should be as important as going to work or eating. The human body is designed to move around, walk, run, and engage in a variety of physical activities. Our body's exercise memory helps us a lot in our old age, when we are considered to fall, and keeps us from falling and breaking bones, and if we fail, it helps us recover quickly.

When exercise is combined with intermittent fasting, it strengthens the muscles of the body, improves strength, consistency, stretching capacity, and stamina, and aids in weight loss in the long run. But there will be more in the following chapters.

Other vitals besides weight should be recorded.

When people begin exercising, it is common for them to gain weight rather than lose it. Most individuals feel that the weight displayed by the weighing scale accurately indicates the body's health. However, this is not the case. When you start exercising, you may not lose weight right once, but your body's fat stores may begin to melt and convert to muscle mass. Muscles have weight as well.

If you have documented the measurements of your body parts, you will be able to spot the difference as soon as it occurs. If you can take measurements of your waist, hips, glutes, and biceps and compare them over time, you will undoubtedly notice the benefits of your efforts. Taking pictures of yourself at the start and end of the program may also help you better understand the impacts of intermittent fasting on your body.

Pay attention to your body.

You may have decided to fast for 16 hours, but if you experience fatigue, excessive hunger, or any other unpleasant effects, pay attention to your body. It is claimed that our bodies are the best coaches for bodily modifications. They can communicate with us by sending out numerous signals at various times to express their demands and necessities.

Begin small.

A 10 to 12-hour fast is also sufficient at first. Later on, if your body adjusts to fasting and you attain your ultimate goals, you can keep adding hours. Even if you are used to fasting for 16 hours, there may be days when you are starving and need to break the fast in 12-13 hours. In any event, pay attention to your body and learn to decipher the signs it sends forth.

Drink plenty of water.

Hydration is essential for optimum health and the efficient functioning of all of our organs. Drink plenty of fluids to stay hydrated, as there are no restrictions on the amount of fluids you can ingest unless you are dry fasting. Though you cannot eat solid foods during fasting, you may drink water, black coffee, unsweetened tea, lemon water, or flavored water. Liquids are required for the cleaning of toxins removed during the fasting phase.

Rest well.

Whether fasting or not, adequate sleep, like food, drink, and the air is critical for human existence. According to certain research, man can survive without food and water for 8 to 21 days, although the maximum time without sleep is 11 days. Sleeping for the required 7 to 9 hours is critical for our bodies to perform at their best. And we never placed a premium on a good night's sleep! When we sleep, our bodies mend and revitalize. We get weary, angry, unable to focus, and lose our feeling of balance and stability when we are sleep deprived for several days at a time. We may also suffer from the cognitive fog. As a result, getting adequate sleep is critical for overall well-being and health.

Please be patient.

Whatever excess weight you have accumulated or health concerns you have are the product of years of neglect and indifference towards your well-being. So, don't expect to lose weight or reverse your diseases immediately if you start intermittent fasting. Changing the circumstances will take time and systematic effort, just as they did to develop over time.

Begin by fasting for a few hours, and then gradually increase your capacity. If you take harsh measures at the start, you will be unable to sustain the fast long enough to realize the benefits. So be patient as you go.

Keeping a journal.

Journaling is an excellent activity to pursue. It aids in retaining memories of good and terrible days, learning and unlearning, and can be referred to at any point in the future. I strongly advise keeping a journal when you begin your intermittent fasting journey. You may keep track of your weight, measurements, fasting schedules, eating windows, physical activity, and even your menu plan. Over time, you can go back through your journal and decide what changes need to be made, whether your past decisions are still working for you, and so on.

WHAT YOU SHOULD NOT DO

Caffeine overdose.

Deep sleep is critical to the effectiveness of intermittent fasting. You don't want to overstimulate your resting digestive system, and too much caffeine may make you too wired and energetic to sleep naturally. Although black coffee is permitted during fasting, too much caffeine may cause acid reflux.

Non-fasting binging.

Though dieting during the non-fasting time is not advised, binge eating should also be avoided. Binge eating causes an increase in calorie intake, which slows the benefits of intermittent fasting. Our goal should be to eat a variety of foods in suitable amounts.

Do not drink anything but water.

Water at room temperature is the greatest way to stay hydrated throughout Intermittent Fasting. Of course, other non-sweetened, zero-calorie liquids are permitted, but they should be consumed in moderation.

Breaking the fast in the wrong way.

Having big meals or feasting on junk food at the end of the fast will limit the amount of food available at later meals, potentially leading to fewer calorie consumption during the eating phase. This could result in an earlier break of fast the next day, reducing the benefits of fasting.

Major food groups are being omitted.

When fasting, it is highly advised that you incorporate proteins, lipids, and carbs in adequate proportions in your diet and other meal components. Leaving any of these major components will be harmful to overall health and may diminish the benefits of fasting.

Never give up.

"Try again if you don't succeed the first time." Success is never attained on the first try. To obtain outcomes, you must endure, be consistent, and be disciplined. Intermittent fasting is the simplest dieting method, but it is not without challenges. There will be difficulties along the way, and you may not always be successful in achieving your fasting goal. Don't be disheartened if you have to break your fast earlier than planned or if you don't receive the expected outcomes in the time frame you set. Maintain consistency and don't give up. You will undoubtedly see effects when you fast every day for a longer time.

Don't give in to your desires.

Craving for the unbidden is a typical inclination. You may crave your favorite foods and feel unusually hungry when fasting. You may have a sweet tooth. But don't succumb to your desires. Keep your long-term objective of becoming a better version of yourself in mind. You may feel too weak at times due to hunger, and you may crave food. Drink some water if you want to extend your fast. It's possible that your appetite may lessen, and you'll feel satisfied. The requirement for hydration might make us feel hungry and irritable at times.

Limit your television viewing.

What!? Isn't that crazy? However, this is not the case. You read that correctly. Limit the amount of time you spend watching television. This is because we are psychologically predisposed to crave chips and popcorn when watching our favorite movie, show, or sport. The food industry, or the junk food industry, has assaulted us with advertisements that show people feasting on chips or colas while watching television.

Beware! When you binge-watch television, you lose track of what and how much you eat. And anything you had was nothing more than empty calories with no nutritional value. You've loaded yourself with sugar and salt, and your body will have to work extremely hard to rid itself of all the junk you've just poured into it.

When fasting intermittently, especially in the early stages, restrict your television time or watch it with someone cautious not to eat while watching TV. If you have a habit of binging in front of the TV, you will crave junk food, and then if you give in to your cravings, you will lose the benefits of fasting and all your hard work.

However, nothing can succeed if your mind is not in the right place. That is why the next chapter is so crucial to read. It is time for us to introduce you to the power of the mind and the power that it plays in this weight loss journey.

SELF-ASSESSMENT

- Which method do you think will work best for you based on your particular needs, preferences, and unique circumstances? (Example: considering your work hours.)
- But before you dive into a particular type from the ones discussed in this chapter, try the suggested 21-day beginner's program mentioned in Chapter Six to give your body and mind time to get accustomed to IF and to build the right mindset and eating habits.

5

"WHAT THE MIND CAN CONCEIVE, IT CAN ACHIEVE" – THE IMPORTANCE OF MINDSET AND HABIT TO THE SUCCESS OF ANY WEIGHT CONTROL PROGRAM

Could your self-perception influence your success or failure? As per Stanford psychologist Carol Dweck, your ideas influence what you desire and whether or not you get it. Dweck discovered that your thinking significantly impacts your success and achievement. So, precisely what is a mindset?

WHAT EXACTLY IS A MINDSET?

Your mindset is a system of beliefs that influence how you perceive the world and yourself. It has an impact on how you think, experience, and act in any given situation.

Types

There are two primary mindsets, according to Dweck: fixed and growth. If your mindset is set, you think that your abilities are fixed traits that cannot be altered. You may also assume that your talent and intelligence are sufficient for success and that no effort is required.

Conversely, if your mindset is growth-oriented, you feel that your qualities and abilities may be developed over time via hard work and perseverance. People with this mindset do not necessarily believe that anyone can become Einstein and Mozart just by trying. They do, though, believe that if people work hard enough, they can become more intelligent or more gifted.

Mindset Development

So, how do you get your mindset in the first place? Dweck's research indicates two key sources: praising but also labeling, which both begin in infancy. Dweck and her colleagues discovered that children acted substantially depending on the type of praise they got in a landmark research series.

They discovered that giving a youngster personal praise, complimenting their talents, or describing them as "clever" encourages a fixed mentality. It communicates to a child that they either have a skill or they don't, so there is nothing they can do about it.

Process appreciation, on the other hand, stresses the effort made to complete a task. It implies that their success results from their action and strategy, which they can manage and improve over time.

Here's an illustration of how they differ. If your child receives an excellent grade on a math test, you could say, "See, you are good at maths. You received an A on your test." On the other hand, process appreciation could be expressed as follows: "I'm impressed by how carefully you studied for your arithmetic test. You went through the subject numerous times, asked your teacher for help with the difficult problems, and tested yourself on it. That was extremely effective!"

Adults can help their children establish growth mind-sets by rewarding effort rather than results. Adults may help children understand that their dedication, hard work, and passion can lead to progress, learning, and progress now and in the future by concentrating on the process rather than the outcome.

The Influence Your Mindset Has

Your mindset influences how you deal with life's obstacles. A child with a growth mindset has a core need to study and work hard to learn new things. This is a sort of academic success.

These same individuals are more likely to endure in the face of failures as adults. On the other hand, those with fixed attitudes are more prone to give up in the face of adversity. Rather than giving up, adults with a growth mindset see it as a chance to learn and progress.

Dweck states in her work that people with fixed mindsets are always looking for validation to establish their worth not only to others but also to themselves.

I've seen many people obsessed with proving themselves in the class, employment, and relationships. Every circumstance necessitates validation of their intelligence, character, or character. Every situation is examined to see if I will succeed or fail. Will I appear intelligent or stupid? Will my application be accepted or rejected? Will I consider myself a winner or a loser?

What about yourself?

Do you think in terms of fixed or growth? Spend some time reading the following points and deciding which ones you agree with the most:

1. You are born with a specific level of intelligence, which cannot be altered.
2. There isn't much you can do to change your basic abilities and personality, regardless of who you are.

3. People have the ability to change who they are.
4. You can expand your knowledge and boost your IQ.
5. People either have specific talents or do not. Talent for things like music, writing, painting, or athletics cannot be acquired.
6. Developing new talents and abilities can be accomplished through study, hard work, and the practice of new skills.
7. If you mostly agree with assertions 1, 2, and 5, you probably have a fixed mindset. Nevertheless, if you agree with claims 3, 4, and 6, you most likely have a growth attitude.

HOW TO FIX A STUCK MINDSET

While individuals with a fixed mindset may disagree, Dweck indicates that people can change their ideas. This is how:

- Concentrate on the journey. Seeing the significance of your journey is critical when developing a growth mentality. When you're focused on the end product, you miss out on everything else you could be studying along the road.

- Include the word "yet." Including this word in your lexicon communicates that you can conquer any obstacle. If you're having difficulty with a task, tell yourself that you haven't mastered it "yet."
- Take note of your thoughts and ideas. To develop a growth mindset, replace negative thoughts with positive ones.
- Accept challenges. Getting it wrong is one of the most effective methods of learning. So, instead of avoiding obstacles, embrace them.

Everything is literally in your head. What attitude do you need to build to be effective with Intermittent Fasting? How can you alter your thinking so that you can successfully fast? How you think about food and your entire mindset may either set you up for success with intermittent fasting or drag you down into failure. We're going to reveal the psychology of intermittent fasting to you.

INTERMITTENT FASTING'S PSYCHOLOGICAL BARRIERS

Three kinds of thinking could be preventing you from fasting successfully. You must overcome those psychological hurdles and change your way of thinking. Nothing can stop you after you've done it.

Fundamental Beliefs

What are your fundamental beliefs, and how do they influence your life? Your fundamental beliefs are firmly established. They are frequently implanted in children while their minds and personalities are still forming. Core beliefs are how you think about everything, from yourself and other people to the world at large. Core beliefs are mostly subconscious; you may not even realize you have a specific idea about something holding you back because it's just how you think about it.

Core beliefs are formed as a result of parental lessons and life experiences, both as a kid and as an adult. In fact, significant adult experiences can even affect a core notion that was imprinted in a youngster. They are frequently reasonably powerful and deeply ingrained, so changing them may be difficult. On the other hand, identifying and modifying your strong ideas about eating and fasting will help you overcome this psychological barrier, enhancing your success.

How to Change Your Fasting Beliefs

Fasting core ideas that stymie your achievement typically look like this:

- You may believe you don't deserve to reduce weight or be healthy. You may be telling yourself covertly and subconsciously that you deserve to be overweight, unattractive, or ill.
- You could think of fasting as a type of self-starvation that isn't healthy or even dangerous.
- You may have a belief about putting in the work that is impeding your progress. In this day of fast pleasure without much effort, you may assume that if something is difficult to obtain or does not happen soon, you cannot do it.

As strange as it may seem, you may subconsciously assume that losing weight will leave you defenseless. Instead of viewing fasting negatively, shift your perspective by replacing negative thoughts with positive ones. As an example:

- Change your self-deprecating notion that you need to be overweight or unwell to believe that you deserve to be healthy and lose weight. Begin to think that you are worth developing for your own satisfaction and that you love doing so.
- If you feel that fasting is terrible for you, that it corresponds to self-starvation, and that it is

destructive, adjust your mind to believe that fasting is beneficial and that it strengthens you.

- If you believe you can't do anything because it's challenging to obtain or doesn't happen right away, start believing that you can. Believe that if you want something strongly enough, you can get it.
- You are mistaken if you believe that decreasing weight will make you vulnerable. Begin to think that it will make you feel powerful and in control.

These are just a few instances, and you may not have them all. Your perspectives on fasting may differ. The take-home message, though, remains the same. When it comes to intermittent fasting, it is critical to replace negative fundamental beliefs with more positive ones. It will take time for that adjustment to take effect, but once you do, the new beliefs will linger with you and make intermittent fasting feel more pleasant.

Self-Talk

Have you ever noticed yourself chatting to yourself about a personal matter? It could be done silently, in your mind, or out loud. What exactly is self-talk, and how does it influence Intermittent Fasting?

The way you talk to yourself about yourself is referred to as self-talk. This mental dialogue with oneself determines how you see yourself and even influences your emotions. Finally, your behavior is affected by your feelings and internal dialogue. Self-talk is frequently associated with core beliefs. You will need to adjust both your underlying beliefs and your self-talk.

You may be telling yourself these thoughts about yourself without even realizing it. Self-talk occurs frequently and is repeated. It is critical to detect negative self-talk and replace it with positive self-talk so that you do not interfere with your success with Intermittent Fasting.

For instance, you may glance in the mirror and tell yourself that you are unattractive. You will feel horrible about yourself as a result of this. These emotions may result in behavior such as always attempting to stay out of the spotlight and avoid drawing attention to yourself. Another way that negative self-talk might influence your behavior is that you never purchase things you enjoy because you convince yourself you don't look good in them and that people will judge you for wearing them.

You must identify and change the negative self-talk that is going on in your head about your health, appearance, and intermittent fasting. When you notice yourself expressing something harmful to yourself, actively oppose it by replacing it with something good. It may even assist to say this new optimistic thinking out rather than just in your head to give it more strength.

Food Regulations

Food rules influence how you perceive and interact with food. These rules may be taught to you by your parents or picked up from others, including society and the media. These rules aren't inherently good or evil; they simply are, yet they can be correct or incorrect.

Consider some of the typical diets available as an example of a dietary rule. Consider the low-carbohydrate diet. Those who adhere to low-carb diets have the power of not eating carbs because they believe and persuade themselves that carbohydrates are detrimental to them. This could be true or false. Carbohydrates can't be good or bad.

However, just because individuals feel better and lose weight does not mean that carbs are unhealthy. They are a kind of fuel for your body; however, if these people lose weight while on a low-carb diet, it supports their idea that carbs are bad.

To be successful, you must first discover any existing food regulations. Once you've recognized them, you must examine them to see whether they are assisting you or hindering you. Food regulations may be impeding your health and weight loss goals; they may also be impeding your success with Intermittent Fasting.

This process, once again, revolves around challenging and changing attitudes and self-talk regarding these norms. After all, you wouldn't have them if you didn't believe in their purpose.

How to Modify Food Regulations

Some standard food rules that may impede you include:

- Maybe you think breakfast is the most important meal of the day since that's what you were taught as a youngster and what society has always told you.
- You may believe that you must eat when others do.
- Maybe you believe that eating and socializing, whether on a date, with friends, or at a function, are inexorably intertwined and that these circumstances must include food.
- You may believe that refusing food is terribly impolite. These are examples of how food restrictions that aren't always true make intermittent fasting practically impossible. You

must transform them by challenging your thinking about them.

- If your food rule is that you must always have breakfast because you believe it is the most important meal of the day, recognize that this is not true and is not benefiting you. Decide only to follow food guidelines that will benefit you.
- If you believe you have to eat when other people eat, decide you have power over what you eat when you eat, and where you eat.
- If you cannot separate eating and socializing, consider how much that link limits your social possibilities to only situations and places where food is accessible. Food isn't the point of socializing; spending time with others is. Your options will also expand.
- Do you believe that refusing food is impolite? Recognize that feeling forced to eat food supplied to you does not benefit you and may harm your health. Understand that when said adequately, folks have no reason to be upset when you say, "Thank you very much."

These are just a few examples of unnecessary meal regulations and how to change them. Your dietary rules may alter, but the procedure remains the same. Identify the regulations, then modify your belief about them and how you talk to yourself about them. Experience fewer difficulties and higher results with intermittent fasting.

How to Overcome Emotional Eating

Emotional eating habits are a psychological and emotional barrier that must be overcome in order to fast without feeling unpleasant. You're on the right track if you picture someone crying and eating a giant tub of ice cream after a breakup. If you eat to fulfill your emotions, fasting becomes a daily battle, and you run the risk of succumbing to stress.

Emotional eating is when you reach for food in response to your emotions. You're not eating because you're hungry; you're eating because you believe it will make you feel better or because you're attempting to feel comfortable in the face of bad feelings. You may even use food as a reward in response to an accomplishment because you believe it will make that accomplishment seem even better. Emotional eating might become so ingrained that you don't even notice you're reacting to emotions with food. How can you tell whether you're an emotional eater? Consider the following questions:

- Do you ever eat when you're not even hungry or when your stomach is already full?

- Do you frequently eat past the point of feeling comfortably full till you feel like you're about to burst?
- Do you ever feel like you can't control yourself regarding food?
- Do you turn to food to make yourself feel better, calm, and soothe yourself when experiencing difficult, unpleasant emotions?
- Do you have a tendency to overeat when you are stressed?
- Do you give food as a reward for accomplishments?
- Do you consider food to be a friend?
- Do you think eating makes you feel safe, similar to how a security blanket makes a toddler feel?

The first step is to recognize that you are eating for emotional fulfillment or comfort. How can you distinguish between emotional hunger and genuine physical hunger? These questions' behavior and thinking are all potential indicators of emotional eating.

- Sudden hunger is often emotional, whereas gradually becoming hungrier is physical.
- You feel the urge to satisfy emotional hunger immediately, although physical hunger can wait a little longer.

- Craving certain, often unhealthy, comfort foods are primarily due to emotional hunger. Because different items sound equally good, a variety of options will satisfy a physical need.
- Physical hunger fades when your stomach is full, but emotional hunger persists even after you feel like you're about to explode.
- When you use food to fill an emotional void or to console yourself, you may experience feelings of shame and guilt. You don't feel guilty about eating since your body is physically hungry.

Determine the Cause

Determine what causes you to eat when you are not physically hungry. You can only begin to replace emotional eating behaviors with healthier habits if you understand what triggers your desire for comfort food. The following are some of the most common causes of emotional eating:

- Stress.
- Negative emotions that you don't want to deal with.
- Growing up with food as a reward from your parents for excellent behavior or

accomplishments or as a source of comfort when you were upset.

- A sense of boredom or emptiness.
- Overeating can occur in social circumstances simply because food is accessible, you are nervous, or someone is pressuring you to overeat.

Emotional Eating Replacement Strategies

- If you feel lonely or unhappy, try reaching out to someone you know may make you feel better. You might also play with a pet or look at anything that makes you joyful.
- Taking a brisk walk or utilizing a stress ball can help alleviate anxiousness or anxiety.
- If you are bored, find something to keep you active or entertained, such as a movie, book, or hobby.
- Relieve tiredness by pampering yourself with anything other than food, such as a hot bath or shower, scented candles, scented body lotion, and so on.
- Deal with unpleasant feelings by confronting them rather than burying them behind the food.

It is critical to develop healthy coping mechanisms to replace emotional eating. It's complicated and unpleasant, but the sooner you learn to confront and deal with your emotions, the sooner you'll be able to control your emotional eating. What works for others may not work for you. Consider and test popular replacement strategies. If they don't work for you, try something else until you find something that will satisfy your emotions and comfort you.

Intermittent Fasting Is Not a Diet

We've said it before, and we'll repeat it because this time, we'll explain why remembering this statement is critical. Intermittent fasting is not a diet and should not be regarded as such. Why? The way you think about and label intermittent fasting influences how you execute it and how successful you are in the short and long run.

Diet is generally associated with slightly negative connotations. When you hear the phrase diet, you probably think of small amounts, monitoring calories, measuring food, and anything light and fat-free.

Do you notice how you already equate dieting with bad conduct and distorted food perceptions? You'll likely identify it with self-deprivation, grumpiness, and excessive desires. You may even imagine diet help commercials for various smoothies, pills, drops, drinks, juicing gadgets, and other products.

If you've ever tried to diet, you know exactly what we're talking about and how painful it can be. For all these reasons, the moment something is classified as a "diet," it becomes something unappealing that you must endure for as little time as possible to achieve drastic short-term benefits.

You don't want to consider intermittent fasting in this way. It will simply make you feel bad about fasting before you even start. When you see something negatively, everything about it appears more difficult and unpleasant than it is. Let's confront the realities for a minute. Intermittent fasting will not be simple, at least not at first. It takes mental fortitude and willpower to alter your body and lifestyle.

That is precisely what intermittent fasting is: a way of life. It would help if you shifted your perspective on fasting from a diet to a way of life. A lifestyle change has more positive implications than dieting. Lifestyle adjustments are considered beneficial and long-term changes that will result in what you desire. In this scenario, it is health, weight loss, and keeping a healthy weight; when you look at something in a more positive light, even the challenging portions that take some getting accustomed to becoming less problematic.

In essence, re-labeling intermittent fasting as a lifestyle rather than a diet aids in changing your mental approach toward it. The appropriate mindset is essential for success. Allow yourself to see intermittent fasting as a lifestyle by letting go of the notion that it is a quick fix that will produce effects in the near term. Crash diets have immediate results but are also generally unhealthy, and the results rarely endure long. You desire long-term benefits from your efforts. You want to be healthier and stay at a healthy weight for the rest of your life. You can only do so if you change your lifestyle, and changing your lifestyle does not happen overnight.

Patience is a virtue that you require.

Be patient with your outcomes. There are several stories on social media and the internet about people who used intermittent fasting to lose a significant amount of weight in a brief period of time. These dramatic fast weight reduction stories only reinforce the notion that fasting is a diet.

You may challenge and change this mental approach by being patient with your outcomes. A healthy weight reduction rate is no more than two pounds each week. Losing more than that is dangerous and may result in consequences such as gaining all of the weight back and then some, as well as health risks. One aspect of considering intermittent fasting as a lifestyle is to accept gradual changes in your body and health.

When you expect to see substantial changes fast, you will be frustrated if they take time, and your resolve to keep going will be weakened. You may make the hasty decision that Intermittent Fasting isn't working and give up before giving your body a chance to adapt and improve.

TIPS

Choose the best fasting time for you.

Given that this is so adjustable, and for you to be successful in this situation, it's best to start by selecting a style that you believe would suit you well. You can follow it in various ways, such as the 16:8 technique or the 20:4 method. The first approach demonstrates how to fast for 16 hours a day and eat inside an 8-hour timeframe. The other method entails fasting for 20 hours and then eating for four hours.

You can select how to begin or end this approach and take a break at anytime between 12 and 8 p.m. In circumstances where breakfast is more important, you should eliminate your evening snacks, and then everything will work much better.

Continue with removing the late-night eating regime.

You can make a significant effect by doing so. Of course, you can eat at night, but then you can avoid consuming many calories because most individuals eat cookies or chips at night. Thus, eating earlier might be beneficial to avoid going to sleep with a full stomach.

Try to keep yourself active most of the time.

Remaining busy can distract you, particularly if you are experiencing hunger. You should avoid consuming excessive foods because of boredom. It may occur when you have nothing to keep your mind active, causing you to believe you are hungry.

You can begin by searching for a different pastime to keep you occupied. The pursuit could be listening to lectures, reading a book, or doing housework. You can also start dancing or exercising out. Maintaining a healthy lifestyle can benefit you, especially during this time, as setting aside 30 minutes to undertake activities will provide a good distraction from always eating.

If you find it challenging to think about food, you should reconsider your current task. This can be accomplished by taking a mental break and altering your everyday routine. In brief, the key issue in this scenario is to keep yourself busy so that thoughts of eating do not linger in your head.

Consume only when necessary.

Fatigue and severe hunger should not be a problem if you follow the 16:8 fasting strategy. However, if you are feeling lightheaded, you should pay attention since your body is attempting to tell you something. For instance, you may have low blood sugar and require food, which is normal.

Furthermore, fasting is reducing some food but not completely starving yourself. So there's no reason to criticize oneself. Instead, choose a protein-rich snack, such as a slice of chicken or a hard-boiled egg, to aid in fat burning. You can then resume your fasting if it is beneficial to you.

Try and listen to your body.

It is critical since you must also keep an eye out for symptoms such as dizziness, weariness, anxiety, and sometimes even stress. These symptoms may indicate that your body is in famine mode and requires sustenance. Also, if you start feeling more relaxed than usual, it's an indication that you should break your fast. You can breach your fast if you frequently experience this.

It would benefit you if you were patient because your body will likely take some time to adjust to fasting, and you may feel hungrier and weaker than usual. However, there is no need to panic when experiencing these sensations, and if the symptoms persist, such as dizziness, you can abandon the diet and find something that can aid you to fit your criteria. Overall, no amount of money can be worth getting sick for.

Limit the number of calories you consume.

You can minimize your calorie consumption, which means that when fasting, you should consume less than 1200 calories. You should limit your consumption during the fasting time since, if you want to maintain a healthy lifestyle, you should try it and see if it works for you. When you slow your metabolism too much, you may lose muscle mass rather than gain it.

Give it some time.

The most important thing you should do is set up a time for Intermittent Fasting. You will not wake up one day and discover that you have lost some weight. No, it may take some time. On the other hand, extreme weight reduction will be observed if you give it some time.

Your body may need some time to adjust, and in this situation, your mental processes may need time to form a habit. If you decide to try intermittent fasting, give it a month before deciding whether or not to continue.

Make changes to your fitness program.

You can exercise while fasting but must be cautious of your motions and timing. You can begin by exercising early, when you may have more energy.

This chapter told you that intermittent fasting is not something that should not be taken seriously and that it has been created to help you determine your health levels and the lifestyle you need to adopt to lose weight at 50. Now that you have all the information you need, we continue to the following chapter, which explains in detail the meal planning process, and what you have to consume.

SELF-ASSESSMENT

- What habits have you formed through the years that you think are now keeping you from realizing your health goals? Do you think you can use the techniques you learned in this chapter to turn them into better habits?
- Conversely, what good habits do you already have that are conducive to your weight-loss objectives?

6

21-DAY FAST MEAL PLAN

With so many different intermittent fasting alternatives available, making a decision can be difficult. We have examined why the Mediterranean diet is the healthiest diet for fasting and non-fasting days. The 16:8 intermittent fasting diet is the most recommended diet for women over 45. Therefore combining these two best options provides the most benefits for women.

The most accessible approach to begin is to have firm ideas for what to eat on fasting and ordinary days. We have created 21 daily food plans for non-fasting and fasting days. But first, let's see why meal planning is important in this case.

THE IMPORTANCE OF MEAL PLANNING

What is meal planning?

- Meal planning is simply planning and writing down your meals for the week ahead of time.
- Make plans for yourself or your family.
- Plan healthful meals and at least one night out. For instance, plan the snacks and dinner options for the upcoming week every Sunday.
- Meal planning can be as accessible or as strict as you like!
- It makes no difference what you plan as long as you are careful and mindful! The idea is not to start from scratch with every meal.

There are numerous reasons why I believe meal planning and meal prepping are beneficial. Still, I think they all fall into three categories: saving time, cutting costs, and having greater control over your food options.

Saving Time

This is the most enticing reason for me. Personally, I love doing things that help me save time. A lot of people need more time than others. Everyone is unique, and everyone's needs are unique.

When you start meal planning, attempt to find one meal where you genuinely need time for something else, and then start planning your meals according to it.

Add additional minutes even on your busiest days by making meals ready to go or by designing very simple, quick dinners that the whole family will enjoy. Also, you can easily ensure that you have all the materials on hand ahead of time!

To begin, choose your busiest days and schedule your meals to be the simplest or prepared in advance to benefit you later.

Cutting Costs

As you plan and cook your daily meals, you are almost certainly saving money on each meal compared to buying the same type of meal at a restaurant.

Furthermore, meal planning can help you decrease food waste, which can save you money on your shopping cost in the long term. While it may be hard to eliminate all waste, some simple planning processes can significantly reduce food loss.

Simply eating leftovers or setting aside a day to consume leftovers is an intelligent way to reduce food waste (and thus save money).

Control Over What You Consume

Everyone is unique, and everyone's needs are unique. Instead of grabbing something at the last minute, planning allows you to make sensible choices about your personal food and exercise demands.

More on How Meal Planning Can Help You Gain Control Over Your Food

Eating the appropriate amount for you.

When you're overly hungry, way too happy to eat, or simply using a various size spoon, you can obtain completely varying/random portion amounts on the plate. Planning but also pre-portioning your food can guarantee that your efforts result in the number of servings you intended. Furthermore, having everything all portioned out for you might be very convenient. If that's not your thing, try a buffet-style meal prep instead!

Maintaining accountability to the past.

If you created the meal and pre-portioned it into immaculate bowls with later you in mind, you're kicking yourself in the buttocks if you don't eat it. Planning and cooking your meals gives you extra motivation to eat the tasty foods you've previously designed and prepared. I'll eat anything if it's already made!

You'll have more say over your options.

If you have specific dietary goals, planning meals in advance can make it much easier to fit them into your routine. It could even be as simple as deciding on a meal to cook or eat, preventing you from ordering food and wasting additional money. In either case, making your decisions ahead of time increases your chances of sticking with them when the time comes.

THE FOOD

It is not a secret that the word "fasting" conjures up ideas of death and destruction, yet intermittent Fasting (IF) has made a commotion in the dieting world. Weight loss and improved blood sugar levels have been demonstrated in a vast number of research. No wonder everyone and their aunt seem to be on board with intermittent fasting these days. Perhaps the lack of dietary restrictions is what attracts people. There are certain restrictions on when you can eat, but there are none on what you can eat in general.

To assist you, we've compiled a list of the best foods to include in your intermittent fasting lifestyle. Balanced food consumption is vital for losing weight, having good energy levels, and trying to keep up with intermittent fasting when there are no specific restrictions or limits on the types or quantities of food that may be ingested.

If you want to lose weight, focus on nutrient-dense foods like fruits, vegetables, whole grains, nuts, seeds, legumes, dairy, and lean meats. In other words, if you eat a lot of the following foods, you will avoid being enraged because you are hungry while fasting. Don't hesitate to get in touch with a health professional before making significant dietary changes to ensure that you make the best decision for yourself and your health.

Food to Consume

Water

Even though it isn't technically a meal, it is essential for living the Intermittent Fasting lifestyle. Drinking enough water is critical for the health of nearly every major organ in your body. It would be foolish to leave this out of your fasting routine.

To put it bluntly, your organs are critical for just remaining alive. Each person's water consumption varies according to gender, weight, height, activity level, and climate.

Dehydration, manifested by dark yellow urine, can cause headaches, fatigue, and lightheadedness, among other symptoms. On the other hand, the color of your urination is an excellent predictor. You want it to be a light golden color at all times.

When you combine it with a limited food source, you have a recipe for disaster - or, at the very least, extraordinarily dark urine - waiting to happen. Water can be more fascinating by squeezing fresh lemon juice, some cucumber slices, or mint leaves.

Seafood

It is sufficient to consume one to three 4-ounce pieces of fish every week. In addition to being an excellent source of healthy fats and protein, it also contains considerable amounts of vitamin D. If you eat at specific times, don't you want to get the most nutritional bang for your buck when you eat something tasty? There are so many ways to prepare fish that you will never be bored.

Avocados

It may appear contradictory to consume the fruit with the highest calorie content while wanting to lose weight. Avocados, though, have many benefits and will keep you full even during the most stringent fasting periods due to their high unsaturated fat content. According to studies (Rosenberg, 2022), unsaturated fats may keep the body satisfied even when you're not hungry. Your organs and tissues ensure that your body has enough nourishment and does not enter emergency hunger mode.

Even though you may feel a bit hungry throughout your fasting phase, unsaturated fats aid in keeping these signs going for a more extended period. For instance, eating half an avocado for lunch can make you feel satiated for up to three hours longer than if you didn't consume that green, mushy gem.

Cruciferous Vegetables

Fiber-rich foods should be ingested at regular intervals to maintain your routine and keep your poop factory working smoothly at all times. Adding fiber may also improve digestion, which is helpful if you cannot eat for the next 16 hours. Fiber, a crucial part of our diet, is abundant in Brussel sprouts, cauliflower, and broccoli. Cruciferous veggies may also reduce your risk of developing cancer.

More information regarding anticancer foods is available below:

- Broccoli - High in sulforaphane, rich with antioxidant properties.
- Carrots - High in antioxidants that promote cancer reduction.

- Beans - High in fiber.
- Berries - High in anthocyanins and several more antioxidant properties.
- Cinnamon - The extract decreases cancer cells.
- Nuts - Rich in selenium that lowers cancer.
- Olive oil - Health benefits that fight cancer.
- Turmeric - Has cumin, an infamous anticancer compound.
- Citrus Fruits - Large amounts of vitamin C.
- Flaxseed - Decrease cancer growth due to high levels of fiber.
- Tomatoes - Have lycopene, rich in anticancer properties.
- Garlic - Has allicin, a compound that kills cancer cells.
- Fatty Fish - High amounts of vitamin D and omega-three fatty acids.

Potatoes

Not even all white foods are bad for your health. Potatoes, for example, were proven to be among the most nutritious foods available. One study (Rosenberg, 2022) revealed that incorporating potatoes into a healthy diet may help with weight loss. Please keep in mind that french fries and potato chips do not count!

Beans and Legumes

Food, specifically its carbs, provides the energy required for physical activity. It is not recommended that you carbohydrate-load excessively, but adding some low-calorie carbohydrates to your diet, such as lentils and beans, wouldn't hurt. This may help you stay awake and attentive during your fasting phase. If you live the IF lifestyle, your favorite chili ingredient could become your best friend.

You know what the tiny organisms in your intestines prefer to eat, don't you? Probiotics are helpful bacteria that aid in the correct functioning of the body. Furthermore, meals including black beans, lentils, chickpeas, and peas have been shown to help people lose weight even when calorie intake is not reduced.

It is critical to maintain consistency and variety. That means that they are not satisfied when they are hungry. You may have unpleasant side effects such as constipation when upset stomach upset. Increase your diet of probiotic-rich foods like kombucha, kefir, and sauerkraut to help relieve gut pain.

Whole Grains

Intermittent fasting and carbohydrate consumption appear to fall into two fundamentally different categories. You'll be relieved to learn that, contrary to popular belief, this isn't always the case. Whole grains are abundant in fiber and protein, so a small amount will keep you full for a long time. So, step outside your comfort zone and look for a whole-grain paradise made of millet, farro, spelt, bulgur, Kamut, quinoa, freekeh, or sorghum grains.

Berries

These components form the basis of your favorite smoothies and are high in helpful nutrients, and that's not even the most incredible part. Over the past 14 years, researchers showed that people who consumed a high concentration of flavonoids, such as those found in strawberries and blueberries, had lower increases in body mass index (BMI) than those who did not eat berries.

Eggs

A large egg contains 6.24 grams of protein and can be made in minutes. Furthermore, getting as many proteins as possible is critical for remaining full and building muscle, especially when eating fewer calories. According to the findings, males who ate breakfast eggs instead of a bagel in the morning were substantially less hungry and ingested significantly less over the day. So, if you're looking for something else to do throughout your fasting period, why not hard boil some eggs and turn them into a meal? Then you'll be able to eat them when the time arises.

Seeds and Nuts

While nuts include more calories than other foods, they deliver beneficial fats that other snacks do not. Furthermore, if you're concerned about calories, don't be! A 1-ounce serving of almonds (equal to 23 nuts) contains 20% fewer calories than the labeled serving size. According to the study's findings (Rosenberg, 2022), chewing does not entirely break down the cell walls of almonds. This leaves some nuts undamaged, which means your body does not absorb them during digestion. As a result, if you eat almonds, they may not play as significant a role in your daily caloric intake as you previously thought.

Foods to Avoid

If you're on an intermittent fasting regimen, there are a few foods you should avoid completely.

- You should avoid foods that are high in calories and high in sugar, fat, and salt, among other things. They will not satisfy your hunger after a fast and may make you feel even more hungry. They are also low in nutritional value.

- If you want to promote a balanced intermittent eating program, avoid the following foods: popcorn toasted in the microwave, snacks, especially chips, and anything fried in seed oils.

You should also avoid meals that have a lot of added sugar. Sugar in processed foods and beverages has no nutritional value and primarily consists of sweet, empty calories, which is the reverse of what you want if you fast on occasion. Because sugar metabolizes so rapidly, you will become hungry. If you practice intermittent fasting, you should avoid the following sweet foods:

- Cookies
- Desserts, especially cakes
- Optional condiments including ketchup and barbecue sauce
- A fruit juice glass
- High-sugar cereals and granola

CAFO meat

CAFO, or Concentrated Animal Feeding Operations, is a mark you do not want to see in your fridge or freezer. That is because the animals from which the meat is produced and later sold under their name are kept in harmful conditions. It can also adopt multiple infections and diseases before reaching your dining table.

What exactly are poisoned vegetables?

Salad veggies are poisoned or infected with bacteria such as E. coli and salmonella due to the heavy use of chemical fertilizers and pesticides and the mixing of untreated sewage water with irrigation water.

Nowadays, there are organically grown, organic veggies available in markets. Organic veggies and fruits may cost a little more, but the money is well spent because they provide more nutritional enrichment than their chemically and artificially cultivated rivals.

21-DAY MEAL PLAN (REPEAT FOR 3 WEEKS)

DAY 1

Breakfast: Smoothie (recipe later on).
Snack: 1 ounce of almonds, walnuts, pecans, macadamias, etc.
Lunch: Chicken or fish curry (4 servings) and a 1/2 of rice.
Four chicken breasts or fish fillets.
One tablespoon of extra virgin olive oil.
One tbsp of mustard.
Two sweet peppers in strips.
1-inch grated ginger.
Two cloves of garlic.

Two medium onions in squares.
Six medium tomatoes, diced.
Half cup unsweetened coconut milk.
Salt to taste.
Curry powder to taste.
Vegetables:
One cup of cauliflower.
One cup of diced zucchini.
One cup of spinach.

Preparation: The protein is prepared in a grilled pan, seasoned with salt to taste. The sauce is prepared separately and then added to the protein — Steamed or boiled vegetables as accompaniments.

DAY 2

Breakfast: Vegetable omelet (1 egg and two egg whites) 1 slice of Ezequiel bread
Snack: Dip with carrot or celery (later on).
Lunch: Chicken breast or salmon with boiled broccoli, chopped vegetables (4 servings), and a 1/2 of rice.
Four boneless chicken breasts o salmon pieces.
One tablespoon of extra virgin olive oil.
Three cloves of crushed garlic.

1 tbsp of crushed parsley.

(Combine everything and marinate the chicken. Then prepare it on the grill).

Vegetables:

One chopped eggplant.

1 tsp salt

Four tablespoons of extra virgin olive oil. - 2 diced zucchini.

Two red peppers in squares.

Two medium onions in squares.

Four crushed garlic cloves.

Two diced tomatoes.

1/4 cup of parsley.

Salt and fresh pepper to taste.

Broccoli: 2 medium heads of boiled broccoli, with salt to taste.

DAY 3

Breakfast: Smoothie

Snack: ¼ of a large avocado chopped to dip with carrots or celery

Lunch: Baked salmon with vegetables (4 servings) and a medium baked potato.

Salmon:

3 tbsp dill.

Four tablespoons of olive oil. - Fresh salmon.

Salt to taste.

Vegetables:

One red bell pepper in strips.

One yellow paprika in strips.

Three tablespoons of extra virgin olive oil. - 2 heads of broccoli.

Sea salt to taste

(Cook the vegetables in a wok).

DAY 4

Breakfast: Vegetable omelet (1 egg and two egg whites), one slice of Ezequiel bread

Snack: Watermelon with a splash of lemon juice and a pinch of salt

Lunch: Meat with vegetables (serves 4) and ¼ cup of rice

Meat:

One tablespoon of extra virgin olive oil.

Three cloves of crushed garlic.

1 tsp fresh black pepper.

1 tbsp of mustard.

Salt and pepper to taste.

Four tenderloin medallions

(The olive oil and other ingredients are combined, and the meat is marinated. It is cooked in a pan with a touch of olive oil to the desired term).

Vegetables:

Four peeled carrots and chopped into strips.

Three stems of celery in strips.

(The vegetables are prepared in the pan with 1 tsp olive oil, sea salt to taste, and a touch of soy sauce).

DAY 5

Breakfast: Acai bowl

Snack: Almonds, walnuts, cashews, peanuts, etc.

Lunch: Chicken and Vegetable Wraps

Chicken:

One cup of extra virgin olive oil.

Two medium onions in strips.

Eight crushed garlic cloves.

Two inches of ginger, crushed or grated - 4 medium-grated carrots.

1 tbsp of fresh pepper.

sea salt to taste

1/4 cup of coriander.

(Vegetables are sautéed. Chicken is boiled and shredded. Vegetables are then added to the chicken).

WRAPS:

16 large romaine lettuce leaves o wraps

Two mashed avocados.

2 cups of spinach.

Lemon.

Preparation: Place the romaine lettuce or wraps on a plate, add the avocado, spinach, and chicken and roll up.

*If you don't want to have breakfast, here is an option you can have for dinner: Soup and boiled egg (Page 6) or a vegetable omelet. (1 egg and two egg whites).

RECIPES:

SOUPS OR CREAMS

Choose the vegetable of your choice, zucchini, mushrooms, cauliflower, broccoli, leek, tomato, etc.

Two tablespoons of extra virgin olive oil.

1/2 medium onion in squares.

1/4 cup of merey.

Two tablespoons of sesame seeds.

1/4 avocado.

Salt and fresh pepper to taste.

1 tbsp of parsley

OLIVE DIP

Two cups of green olives.

One clove of garlic.

One tablespoon of extra virgin olive oil. (blend until creamy).

SPINACH DIP

One tablespoon of extra virgin olive oil.

8 cups of spinach.

One clove of garlic.

(The spinach is sautéed for 5 minutes with a little bit of olive oil. It is blended by adding olive oil).

.   .   .

SMOOTHIE

1 cup of berries, pineapple, banana, kiwi, or the fruit of your choice

1 tbsp peanut or almond butter.

1 tbsp of chia seeds.

Two raw walnuts.

1 inch of ginger.

1/4 avocado.

1/2 cup of almond milk.

1/2 cup of water or ice.

I hope that you loved the information presented in this chapter. I hope that you also clearly understand what the recipes should look like and what you should consume or prepare. The next chapter addresses the most common concerns about intermittent fasting. Let's learn everything there is regarding it.

SELF- ASSESSMENT

You've learned the importance of meal planning and how to plan meals with weight loss in mind. You also have two suggested meal plans to get started. Source the food items you need based on the plan of your choice; prepare your body and mind, and start your IF journey.

7

INTERMITTENT FASTING FAQ

There is a lot of contradicting information about intermittent fasting out there. Some of that information is correct, some is misleading, and some is entirely incorrect. We'll debunk some fasting fallacies and address the most frequently asked fasting questions.

MYTHS ABOUT INTERMITTENT FASTING

Myths about intermittent fasting aren't usually related to abstention from food. Some myths that cause you to doubt fasting are common meal myths, while others are antiquated or plain false.

Skipping breakfast will cause you weight gain.

This myth is based on the belief that breakfast is the day's most important meal and that you must break your overnight fast first thing in the morning. Why do people believe that skipping breakfast will cause you to gain weight?

There is a widespread belief that skipping 'the most important meal of the day can cause you to become insatiably hungry and experience tremendous cravings, resulting in overeating or grabbing out unhealthy snacks, hence weight gain.

Studies have shown that eating breakfast improves performance and may result in steady weight loss over time. However, a considerable number of people have found success with weight loss through intermittent fasting, which frequently means skipping breakfast. So, the jury is still out on whether breakfast is the most important meal of the day, and no evidence certifies that skipping it harms your weight.

Remember: Everyone is unique and will react differently to similar events. Skipping breakfast may have little effect on one person, but it may cause issues for the next. Recognizing that uniqueness introduces unpredictability into the equation and being conscious of your personal needs is critical.

Eating frequently boosts your metabolism.

Everyone has heard that eating numerous smaller meals more regularly is preferable to eating three larger meals less frequently. This claim is based on the premise that eating regularly stimulates your metabolism and makes it more efficient at burning fat. The flip side of this myth is that eating less frequently may reduce your metabolism, resulting in weight gain.

So, if intermittent fasting slows metabolism, why are there many people trying to lose weight with it? Well, keep in mind that individual diversity plays a role in everything. Your particular needs will influence what type of meal frequency works best for you. However, there is a trend that reveals this myth to be false.

Eating frequently promotes weight loss.

Why might meal frequency affect weight loss or weight gain if it doesn't necessarily raise or slow your metabolism? This is another issue of personal choice and your body's specialized needs vs. a claim being true for everyone.

Fasting causes your body to go into starvation mode.

This is a prevalent misconception regarding fasting and is frequently cited as an argument against it. According to the hypothesis, going without food puts you into starvation mode, where your metabolism slows to a crawl to support just vital processes, making fat burning difficult or practically impossible.

When fasting for extended periods of time (think days, not hours), your metabolism may naturally slow down. This is a natural survival response after going days without nutrition. But, when you do not consume food for an extended period of time, your body goes into ketosis mode. This means that your fat or ketones are broken down into energy when glucose is absent. This may, in fact, temporarily boost your metabolism.

Eating more frequently keeps hunger at bay.

It is believed that eating smaller meals more frequently helps to reduce severe hunger and food cravings. Individuality will influence the outcome in this scenario as well.

It may not be accurate for everyone, but it may be true for some. Because of this variation, some people find fasting for more extended periods easier than others. Their bodies may be better at working for extended periods without triggering hunger. Others may find it more challenging to adopt intermittent fasting because their bodies are the polar opposite.

Overeating is a result of Intermittent Fasting.

This is definitely not true. At least not for every single person. Some people may compensate for their fasting phase by overeating in terms of quantity or calories during their eating window. That's not always the case, and by managing your intake as well as eating a good, balanced diet, you may train your body to cycle between fasting and eating. When your body adjusts, your hunger pangs should go away, as should the desire to compensate.

Intermittent fasting is harmful.

Only a medical specialist can tell you whether or not intermittent fasting is healthy for you. Intermittent fasting has varied effects on different people. Have this on your mind. On the other hand, fasting has been linked to several health benefits. This alone disproves the notion that it is generally unhealthy.

INTERMITTENT FASTING: FREQUENTLY ASKED QUESTIONS

We've examined a range of what you need to know and want to know about intermittent fasting. Many frequently asked issues have been addressed; however, there are still a few to be managed.

Should You Do Anything Different as a Woman?

While both men and women can benefit from intermittent fasting, some fasting strategies are more suited to women. Men can generally fast for more extended periods of time than women, who do better with shorter fasts. Women who fast on a regular or daily basis may wish to explore a 14:10 schedule rather than a 16:8 or greater schedule.

Similarly, if you choose a fasting strategy with fasting days and normal days, women tend to perform better with the 5:2 diet than other approaches such as Alternate Day Fasting or even the East Stop Eat method.

One of the reasons women benefit from shorter fasting intervals is that fasting alters their feminine hormones. The longer you fast, the more your hormones are influenced. As a result, fasting for a shorter period of time has less of an effect on your hormones.

How long and how frequently should you fast?

Fasting offers health benefits but is not a cure-all if you are not healthy. The length and regularity of your fasting will be determined by your specific goals as well as your current health and weight. If you are not in good health, fasting may not be a great idea until you have enhanced your health. If you start an intermittent fasting regimen without consulting your doctor, you may do more harm than good.

Weight influences the frequency of Intermittent Fasting. The length of your fast will be determined by the type of fasting plan you are participating in as well as your gender. If you are holding more weight, you may be able to fast more regularly than someone who does not have the same level of body fat. It is also critical that your eating window allows you to consume enough calories to meet your demands and goals.

For example, if you are a light eater who struggles to consume meals that suit your needs in a short amount of time, fasting on a 20:4 schedule will not work for you.

What can you drink while fasting?

When it comes to something to drink when fasting, water is your best bet. However, you can drink almost any beverage that contains no or significantly no calories. Drinks sweetened with non-nutritive sugar substitutes are a good choice for calorie-free liquids. But, you should proceed with caution because it has been hypothesized that sugar substitutes may negatively influence the microorganisms in your gut, which may alter your metabolism. Here are some options for quenching your thirst:

- Water.
- Black coffee with artificial sweetener or no sugar.
- Tea with no sugar or milk.
- Zero-calorie carbonated beverages and sugar-free sports drinks.

What about cream and milk in coffee and tea?

When you fast, your body enters ketosis, which is a clever phrase for a fat-burning state. Adding carbohydrates may cause you to break your fast. As a result, adding milk and cream may have a negative effect. Because it has more fat than milk, cream is a better choice. Because they are fats and not carbohydrates, adding healthy fats to your coffee or tea, such as coconut oil or a tiny quantity of butter, may not cause you to break your fast.

How do you know when you are in a fasted state?

A blood and breath ketosis meter is the only way to determine if you are in ketosis. However, after around 12 hours of fasting, your body should enter ketosis and begin burning fat. This time range may vary slightly depending on your metabolism. By eight hours following your last meal, your food should have completed the digestion and absorption process. After this period, your body will begin to burn stored glycogen for energy. By 12 hours, those stores should be depleted, and fat-burning should begin.

What is the scientific basis for Intermittent Fasting?

Fasting causes our bodies to enter a mildly stressed state known as hormesis. Our cells adjust during hormesis, which may increase fat burning, metabolic rate, and other physiological functions.

Most of the time, individuals consume fewer total calories than non-fasters, resulting in weight loss. This could be due to a variety of individual characteristics, or it could simply be that a limited eating window suppresses certain habits, such as late-night snacking.

Is one intermittent fasting approach more effective than another?

Some people limit their meals to an 8-hour window, but others alternate between an entire day of fasting and a day of normal eating. There is no one way of intermittent fasting that has been shown to be more successful than another.

Fasting, like regular eating habits, should be tailored to the individual and their lifestyle. Some people can sustain genuine fasting during the day, while others function better when they eat more regularly.

8

TROUBLESHOOTING - WHEN YOUR IF EXPERIENCE ISN'T AS PLEASANT AS YOU HOPED FOR

The first thing we need to clear up is that fasting will not cause you to starve to death. This fear-based negative thinking acts as a self-fulfilling prophecy. The human body has evolved to withstand fasting spells. If you're two minutes into a fast, hungry, convinced yourself it's hopeless, and fixated with your next meal, you're not going to get anywhere.

While you may benefit from intermittent fasting in terms of weight loss, enhanced hormone function, and better sleep, you may also experience a few adverse effects of fasting. When it is certain that you may feel hungry at some point while fasting, intermittent fasting tiredness may be the second most common side effect.

When intermittent fasting weariness sets in, it's tempting to give up and grab your favorite food to comfort the body and mind. So, how can we avoid this weariness while also preventing hunger strikes?

CONSUME WATER

While it may be tempting to simply drink a cup of strong coffee and wake up your body and mind, this will only treat the symptom of your fasting weariness, not the reason. According to studies, even slight dehydration can make you feel weary, whether you're genuinely tired or not.

Dehydration causes a reduction in blood pressure, which reduces blood supply to the brain. You also have a decrease in blood volume, making your heart work harder to pump nutrients, oxygen, and hydration to the various cells. All of this contributes to exhaustion and sleepiness.

You may notice usual hunger signs such as rumbling or an empty stomach. To make matters worse, mild dehydration signs frequently resemble hunger feelings. Consider whether you need a snack or just a drink of water.

We could go on and on about the advantages of drinking water, especially during intermittent fasting when water consumption is reduced due to fewer meals taken. One thing is sure: If you stay hydrated, you will avoid most intermittent fasting adverse effects and feel healthier and more energized.

CONSUME MORE FOOD

Following the preceding tip about assessing your diet, you may conclude that you need to eat more nutritious meals to get the necessary nutrients. This is especially true if you have a more active lifestyle, such as working out or having a more mobile job. You could not be getting enough calories to keep your energy levels up.

Even if your objective for intermittent fasting is to lose weight, you should not sacrifice your health!

If you believe that not eating enough is causing your intermittent fasting fatigue, try shortening your fasting window to accommodate a few nutritious snacks or a small healthy meal. You might also consider intermittent fasting supplements to increase your vitamin and mineral intake.

CONSUME LESS FOOD

You just said to eat more food! You might feel tempted to binge eat after your fasting period is over. It all depends. Overeating is a common intermittent fasting pitfall, especially for new intermittent fasters.

However, doing so may compromise your weight loss goals and make you feel dull or weary after your large meal.

A little tiredness after a meal is normal, especially if you consume a large meal or foods heavy in carbohydrates. It causes your blood sugar to spike quickly after eating and then plunges, resulting in a blood sugar "crash."

Break your fast with a smaller meal, preferably with fewer carbs, to reduce post-meal weariness. You may try yogurt, bone broth, or a salad of leafy green vegetables.

MAKE A CUP OF COFFEE

Sometimes all you need is a short boost of energy and focus. When everything else fails, coffee can come to your rescue. Fortunately, black coffee is one of the few drinks you can consume when fasting. However, there should be no sugar or cream.

Stick to the recommended 2 – 3 cups of coffee per day and avoid coffee at night. You don't want it to disrupt your excellent night's sleep and make you exhausted the next day.

9

EXERCISING WHILE INTERMITTENT FASTING - IS IT A GOOD IDEA?

The human body is designed in such a way that it can undertake numerous physically demanding tasks throughout the day, every day. Our forefathers, who were hunters and gatherers, would travel the brush all day gathering food and running after animals to hunt them for food.

These activities kept them physically busy at all times. However, with the emergence of comfort products during the previous 4-5 decades, physical activity in daily life has decreased dramatically. We hardly do any physical work.

The majority of items are accessible with the press of a button. This has made us sluggish and less active, so we must make time for workouts and exercise to maintain our bodies active and attentive.

Workouts are highly important for ladies in the peri-menopausal or menopausal stages. These are women between the ages of 40 and 45. Many of these ladies may have rarely exercised when they were younger because working out wasn't considered cool.

EXERCISE IS REALLY IMPORTANT FOR MENOPAUSAL WOMEN.

As described in earlier chapters, as women over 40 enter the perimenopausal and later menopausal stages of their lives, they experience many unpleasant symptoms such as hot flashes, inflammation, bone weakness and loss of muscle tone, heart disease, and so on.

The most serious of these is weight gain in the abdominal area, which is the core cause of many later-onset diseases. However, it is crucial to note that just as each woman is unique, so is her menopause experience. Some people may endure severe symptoms, while others find the shift simple. Whatever the case, this is the period in your life when taking care of yourself is critical.

Implementing time for self-care and making minor lifestyle modifications might help you manage the changes in your body. Incorporating little workout sessions into your everyday routine is one such modification. Here are a few reasons why you should include an exercise plan into your daily routine:

Improves your mood.

Exercising increases the production of endorphins, the brain's feel-good chemicals. These endorphins aid in the relief of stress and the reduction of overall tension. It improves your mood and lowers your risk of depression and cognitive deterioration. Better mental health also promotes higher self-esteem and enhances sleep quality.

Stops excessive weight gain.

Most of the population, particularly women, struggle with a middle-age weight increase. This is due to a combination of internal and environmental causes.

A woman in her 40s or 50s usually has grown-up or adolescent children, which means that the energy she expended running around toddlers and kids is no longer being used. She is in a much better place professionally and socially; therefore, there may be an excess of energy devoted to those two aspects of her life.

Furthermore, her metabolism rates decrease as she ages and her body changes. All of these factors contribute to weight gain, which can be minimized or avoided to some extent by leading an active lifestyle and incorporating some mild exercise into the routine.

Bones and muscles are strengthened.

The capacity of the bones to hold calcium decreases with age and the onset of menopause, making the bones brittle in the long term and ultimately leading to the onset of osteoporosis. Muscles begin to lose bulk and sag as well. Regular exercise has been shown to be particularly efficient in bone and muscle building. It reduces the pace of bone loss, lowering the risk of fractures.

Reduces the likelihood of developing cancer and other disorders.

As outlined in the metabolism chapter, regular exercise keeps the body in an anabolic or building state. It prevents uncontrolled cell growth. Exercise also helps to maintain a healthy body weight, which protects against diseases such as breast, colon, and endometrial cancer.

FASTING AND EXERCISE

Many health doctors advise exercising only after a couple of hours of eating a nutritious meal. However, several studies have shown that exercising while fasting is far more beneficial for fat loss. Let us take a closer look at both of these assertions.

After-meal exercise

Many nutritionists recommend eating a carbohydrate-rich pre-workout meal and a protein-rich post-workout meal. The carbohydrate-rich pre-workout meal makes your body have enough energy to do the workout. Because when you exercise, the additional power the body requires is fueled by burning the carbs from the pre-workout meal. As a result, when you exercise after meals, you will feel more energized and will be able to exercise with the appropriate technique. Furthermore, your blood sugar levels will remain stable with a filled stomach, keeping you alert and active; having a proper lunch before a workout is vital for improving endurance training performance.

Exercising while fasting

Many intermittent fasting researchers and proponents recommend exercise throughout the fasting time. According to these organizations, when you work out on an empty stomach, you don't have any carbohydrates to fuel your energy needs.

This encourages cells to delve deeper into fat stores to produce energy for exercise, which may result in higher fat loss than would otherwise occur. However, you should be aware that when you are fasting, your blood glucose level is already lower, and your energy levels may be lower than after eating.

This may produce lightheadedness or dizziness; in extreme cases, you may faint on the exercise floor. Exercising without eating may also be ineffective when building and improving your muscles, even if it does not result in muscle loss.

We saw in the last section that exercising could be done a few hours after meals and even while fasting. So the question is, what should we do now? Which of the two is preferable? Is it better to exercise after meals or on an empty stomach? The answer to this question differs depending on who you ask. Let me share a few factors to think about before making a decision.

Exercise type

The amount of energy required for exercise is determined by the sort of exercise undertaken. The endurance exercises require enough power to maintain appropriate form and performance. If you do high-intensity interval training, your energy requirements will be substantially higher than if you do yoga or meditation.

Exercise schedules

If you plan on doing a longer workout, you may require more energy than your body can offer. In such instances, it is best to consume something before exercising. However, if you want to exercise while fasting, you can schedule your workout just an hour before you break the fast. For example, if you fast for 16 hours and your eating window is 12 noon to 8 p.m., you can schedule your workout at 11 a.m.

Your body is already using stored body fats for energy at this point, and doing it in that state will help you burn more fat. However, exercising beyond eight o'clock is not recommended in the same case. This is because if you exercise after meals, you will burn through all of the carbohydrates in your body within an hour of starting your fast.

Fasting for another 15 hours will be pretty challenging after that. You will have hunger pangs and desires for sweet foods, and if these cravings are not satisfied, you may feel irritable and grumpy. In addition, the body requires nutrition after an exercise to recover. Amino acids, for example, can be utilized to make proteins, whereas carbohydrates can restore your body's glycogen stores.

So, a meal after a workout is significantly more important, yet this does not mean you have to eat right away.
It is strongly advised to eat within two hours of exercising. To summarize the preceding discussion, we can say
that, if feasible, the workout should be arranged an
hour before breaking the fast, followed by a nutrition-
ally dense meal.

RECOMMENDED EXERCISES

Aerobic or cardiovascular exercise

Aerobic exercise works for broad, muscular groups
while keeping your heart rate elevated. It aids in the
loss of excess weight and the maintenance of a healthy
weight. Aerobic exercises that you can begin with
include brisk walking, swimming, cycling, and jogging.
Do it for 10-15 minutes at first, then progressively
increase the time and intensity.

Strength training

A few years ago, many women believed that strength
training was only for guys and that lifting weights
would cause them to bulk out like men. But this is not
the case. Strength exercise strengthens your muscles
and keeps them from losing bulk as you age, saving you
from the risk of osteoporosis. It also protects you from
hip fractures caused by a fall in the restroom in your

golden years. It aids in reducing body fat and effectively burns calories by speeding up your slowing metabolism as menopause approaches. Strength training should be done under the supervision of a certified trainer. Strength training can, however, be done at home with modest weights and resistance bands. Choose weights that will wear you out in 12 repetitions and then gradually increase from there.

Meditation and yoga

Stretching exercises should be performed after each workout when the muscles are more susceptible to stretching. Yoga poses stretch different muscles in your body and provide relief from menopause symptoms such as hot flashes, irritation, and weariness. It also strengthens and stretches the joints. Meditation and deep breathing help to settle your mind and provide a sense of relaxation. This aids in the improvement of your sleep quality.

Zumba and dancing

If completing repetitive sets of exercise isn't your thing, try a dancing class or Zumba. Both disciplines incorporate dance, music, and a lot of cardio moves. The dance works your muscles and increases your flexibility, while the music boosts your spirits.

Gardening and other activities

Working hard in your garden so that a major muscle group, such as the quads, glutes, and core, is worked also counts as a workout. Finally, whatever type of workout you choose, make it a point to perform it an hour before breaking your fast to burn the most fat, and break the fast quickly after the workout to replenish your muscles with critical nutrients.

FINAL WORDS

Intermittent fasting is not a fad diet but rather a way of living, a manner of life. There is no right or wrong way to live. Fasting has been around for as long as people have been. Fasting is encouraged in most cultures and religions around the world for a variety of reasons. On the other hand, fasting for health is a relatively new phenomenon that piqued the interest of many people worldwide, both young and old.

The health benefits of Intermittent fasting are numerous, as we have covered throughout this book, particularly for women in their 40s and 50s who find it difficult to lose weight and face risks from a variety of diseases owing to the hormonal changes in their bodies.

However, each woman is distinct. Her experience with menopause is also one-of-a-kind. Some women may not feel any symptoms, and menopause may appear to be an easy transition. Others may experience symptoms that are so severe that they are unable to function.

In this case, all that can be said is that Intermittent fasting is a lifestyle change rather than a medical treatment. You should attempt it after talking with your doctor and under their supervision. After that, let your bodies have a few days to acclimate to the fasting lifestyle and monitor the changes in your physical and mental well-being.

Listen to your body and notice the changes that occur. If you notice any favorable benefits, continue the intermittent fasting to the best of your ability. However, if you encounter the side effects of intermittent fasting, modify your fasting schedule as necessary to eliminate the side effects.

Furthermore, if you encounter long-term adverse effects from intermittent fasting, it may be a sign that it isn't working for your body. These could be the side effects:

- Extreme hunger
- Nausea
- Irritability

- Headaches
- Exhaustion
- Fainting

If intermittent fasting is making you unhappy, stop doing it. Despite the fact that this manner of eating has been linked to health benefits, there are numerous other things you may do to improve your health that does not include fasting.

A balanced and healthy diet, adequate sleep, regular physical activity, and stress management are far more crucial for overall health.

I've tried to discuss as much as possible about intermittent fasting and its effects on women over the age of 50 without sounding preachy. I hope that the chapters in this book have enriched your life. Good luck and have fun with your new way of life.

REFERENCES

Mindikoglu, A. (2020). Intermittent fasting from dawn to sunset for 30 consecutive days is associated with anticancer proteomic signature and upregulates vital regulatory proteins of glucose and lipid metabolism, circadian clock, DNA repair, cytoskeleton remodeling, immune system, and cognitive function in healthy subjects. Journal of proteomics, 217, 103645.

https://doi.org/10.1016/j.jprot.2020.103645

Colon cancer, nuts, and early onset. UConn Health. (n.d.). Retrieved July 2, 2022, from https://health.uconn.edu/archives/uconn-health-podcast/colon-cancer-nuts-and-early-onset

Patterson, R. E., & Sears, D. D. (2017). Metabolic effects of Intermittent Fasting. Annu Rev Nutr, 37(1), 371-93.

De Cabo, R., & Mattson, M. P. (2019). Effects of intermittent Fasting on health, aging, and disease. New England Journal of Medicine, 381(26), 2541-2551.

Made in the USA
Monee, IL
12 August 2023

40916281R00098